Raise a Puppy

The Essential Guide to Raising and Training Your Puppy

(How to Raise a Puppy to Become an Obedient Well Behaved and Loving Dog)

Eric Upton

Published By **Andrew Zen**

Eric Upton

Raise a Puppy: The Essential Guide to Raising and Training Your Puppy (How to Raise a Puppy to Become an Obedient Well Behaved and Loving Dog)

ISBN 978-1-998927-02-9

No part of this guidebook shall be reproduced in any form without permission in writing from the publisher except in the case of brief quotations embodied in critical articles or reviews.

Legal & Disclaimer

The information contained in this book is not designed to replace or take the place of any form of medicine or professional medical advice. The information in this book has been provided for educational & entertainment purposes only.

The information contained in this book has been compiled from sources deemed reliable, and it is accurate to the best of the Author's knowledge; however, the Author cannot guarantee its accuracy and validity and cannot be held liable for any errors or omissions. Changes are periodically made to this book. You must consult your doctor or get professional medical advice before using any of the suggested remedies, techniques, or information in this book.

Upon using the information contained in this book, you agree to hold harmless the Author from and against any damages, costs, and expenses, including any legal fees potentially resulting from the application of any of the information provided by this guide. This disclaimer applies to any damages or injury caused by the use and application, whether directly or indirectly, of any advice or information presented, whether for breach of contract, tort, negligence, personal injury, criminal intent, or under any other cause of action.

You agree to accept all risks of using the information presented inside this book. You need to consult a professional medical practitioner in order to ensure you are both able and healthy enough to participate in this program.

Table Of Contents

Chapter 1: Before Bringing Your Puppy Home

Bringing a current-day puppy home is a lovable treat for the entire circle of relatives, one that may extensively brighten everyone's day. Since granting a secure and loving domestic for a puppy isn't always any small feat, there are a few subjects to don't forget ahead of time.

Puppies are tiny, defenseless, and an extended manner away from their mom, simply so they need more care and a watchful eye to make sure that they broaden healthfully. You might be a bit crushed and harassed as to how precisely you ought to skip about doing so, and it's best natural that you are feeling this manner. With a few research and cautious making plans, despite the fact that, you'll truely end up a skillful fur-figure proper away.

Can You Afford a Puppy?

Looking at the photograph of proudly owning a dog from an intruder's mindset may not reflect the truth, mainly concerning the expenses. So, earlier than you're making the choice, don't forget all the following prices of getting a puppy and decide whether or not or not you could without a doubt locate the money for one.

Upfront prices

When it entails dogs, the form of prices can variety immensely counting on primary elements: the breed and whether or not or not you're shopping for or adopting. Because a few breeds are unusual or are purchased for specific functions, the initial fee can be quite high; however, there is continuously the choice of adopting a dog from the closest secure haven. The benefit is that, in most instances, you received't in truth pay something—otherwise you'll pay a minimal amount and also you'll be giving a homeless canine a all the time domestic.

Vaccines and microchipping

Another in advance value to take into consideration upon getting a canine is purchasing the necessary vaccines. Depending on what it's already taken, how antique it's far and which season you're in, there may be one-of-a-kind vaccines available, however anyways, it's miles a charge which you must preserve in thoughts. Getting your home dog microchipped is some other vital upfront, one-time charge to expose ownership in case your canine is out of area, and it's a must in case you're ever making plans to excursion remote places. While the ones fees might also to begin with add up considering the reality that they commonly emerge at the identical time, they may be splendid paid as quickly as. It is likewise well really worth citing that adopting a dog from a safe haven can from time to time decrease the preliminary expenses as they have a tendency to already be vaccinated and microchipped.

Bedding, collar and toys

When thinking about preliminary charges, don't overlook that you'll additionally want to shop for a cushty vicinity for the most updated member of your circle of relatives to sleep in. You'll want a collar and leash for at the identical time as you take your dog out for a walk and a few toys to maintain it entertained, particularly even as it's home by myself—this will honestly save you it from ruining your fixtures out of boredom, too. While you're at it, you need to moreover get a call tag collectively with your name and range on it, without a doubt if your furball ends up getting out of place.

Dog meals

Depending on the dimensions and interest diploma of your dog, the amount of food it'll devour may additionally additionally range. On average, a younger, medium-sized dog will undergo 30 kilos of dry canine food in six to 8 weeks. If you pick out to feed your domestic dog raw or home-cooked food, you want to calculate those charges as nicely.

Vet care

Don't neglect to think about commonplace visits to the vet and additionally assume that similar to little babies, puppies moreover will be inclined to get sick and could need to be taken to a vet, that can absolutely upload as an lousy lot as the overall costs of searching after a home canine.

It is vital to keep in mind that dogs require right care and embody their very personal set of charges that you want to be prepared for. Taking a majority of these charges below interest will assist you to nicely budget in your modern-day day family member. And in case you're nonetheless in the choice segment, cautiously reading a number of the ones points can provide you with an idea of whether or not or not you may surely find the cash for a pup or not, in advance than you take on the obligation and come to be getting alarmed with the useful aid of the quantity of fees you want to cowl.

What You Need to Get

Owning a canine isn't always reasonably-priced, in order that's one component you want to take into account earlier than adopting a home dog. And on the equal time as many households can control to pay for to get a canine, only some have greater time on their hands to invest in a modern-day family member. Unlike their tom cat opposite numbers, puppies need lots of interest, specially within the occasion that they're nevertheless in their nurturing segment.

However, in case you expect you have extra money and time for your arms to in the end adopt a puppy, right here's what you want to get earlier than your enjoy to the safe haven.

Dog-proof fence

Canines are surely curious creatures. The proper news is, inside the event that they ever discover their way out, they'll likely be able to have a study the fragrance returned domestic. However, there's masses to fear about past the fence of your home that might seriously injure your canine, and in some severe times, result in its demise.

If you don't have a fence right now, don't convey your canine domestic within the want of maintaining it as a strictly indoor doggy. Even if you walk your dog every morning, you're despite the fact that going to want it to wander approximately for your outdoor for some mild solar exposure, and to provide it extra vicinity to find out and get enough exercising at the same time as no longer having to be on a leash.

Dogs also usually will be predisposed to get bored without trouble, so get right of entry to to the outdoor will allow them to examine your friends and perhaps even chase a few squirrels. Don't fear, it's now not going that they'll trap any of them.

Just ensure you limit your canine's get right of entry to to open regions to sunlight hours, because it will in all likelihood bark at passing pedestrians, which can be annoying on your buddies in the useless of night.

Another motive you want to get a fence is that it lets in your exquisite pal to freely get common relaxation room breaks. This is specifically vital at the same time as it's despite the fact that a home canine; you'll must train it wherein it's good enough to transport potty, in any other case you'll have loads to clean up on a every day basis.

Just consider that getting a fence does not replace taking your canine on a walk. Dogs want to be walked each day for a trade of surroundings, an good enough quantity of workout, and some intellectual stimulation. This additionally enables you bond collectively along with your new domestic dog and offers it a few component to sit up for each day.

Pet gates

Whether you're adopting a extra youthful puppy or selecting a senior canine, you're going to want to maintain the nosy little furball a long way from elements of your home that might be dangerous for it to discover, or every other place that you'd need to keep smooth and tidy. Canines are curious and messy, and any room they access can also moreover additionally grow to be being issue to 3 chewed up gadgets or damaged vases.

There are gates specially designed for pets, but a few are so low that your pup can discover ways to jump over them. Make fantastic the gates you pass for are every immoderate and sturdy enough.

We propose you get the ones installed at multiple entrances; despite the truth that, you shouldn't maintain them closed usually. They may be a notable way to location your canine now not to interrupt you at the same time as you're cooking or consuming. For the first few months, assume your dog to bark and wail at the closed gate. It could be heartbreaking, however in the long run, your dog could have a examine while and wherein it could get proper of access to regions in your house.

The opportunities are endless in relation to where you could set up pet gates, however we would advocate in opposition to overusing them. Dogs count on to be dealt with as a part of the family. If you restriction their get proper of access to to multiple areas for prolonged periods of time, this also limits the time you spend together together together with your canine, that could take a toll on their mental health. Use the gates reasonably, on the equal time as you genuinely want to.

Chew toys

Think of bite toys as pacifiers for toddlers. In their teething section, dogs will both chew on the numerous toys which you provide them, or they'll chunk holes thru your fixtures. There's number one/three alternative.

Chewing for growing puppies is corresponding to an itch that wants to be scratched, and it permits them develop healthy enamel short. However, that's no longer to say that sincerely-grown dogs will save you the use of their chunk toys. Wild dog actually exert pretty a few attempt whilst chewing thru the flesh and bones of their prey—a herbal intuition that canned or dry meals does now not satiate. Because your canine doesn't go out to are in search of for, it wants to find out a few detail else to chew on apart from prey.

Your options are infinite, and options completely depend upon your dog. Most canine, especially dogs, revel in squeaky toys because of the fact they mimic squealing prey. It can also sound ugly, however it's simplest intuition. You'll most likely want to offer your home dog with loads of toys to pick from.

Bigger plush toys may be their desired to once in a while chew on, and moreover use as snuggle pillows when they nap. Bone-original squeaky toys are usually incredible distractions to skip the time, or to revel in some great playtime with you.

If you'll depart your canine unaccompanied for a few hours, the exquisite toy to preserve it entertained with is a rubber bite treat toy, which may be complete of treats that ooze out of the toy even as bit or squeezed. This additionally mimics a searching enjoy, that allows you to keep your dog's instincts satiated, and could, in flip, assist keep your domestic dog properly-behaved.

There are also flavored toys, which double as toothbrushes for your doggy. These toys are especially designed with easy bristles that clean your canine's enamel as it chews at the toy. They're high-quality for a few extra dental care, but don't overlook that they may be capable of't replace an extensive toothbrushing ordinary. Some puppies also are finicky close to cheap rubber that smells artificial. Opt for a flavored toy to make it extra attractive for your canine.

Food and water accessories

You have to invest in some strong and easy-to-clean food and water bowls as soon as you can. Growing puppies have extensive appetites and you need to ensure which you have the right gear reachable to feed them regularly. It's beneficial to get a fairly huge water bowl, too, as all dogs need smooth get right of access to to clean, sparkling water continually.

Furthermore, you want to placed your domestic dog on a food plan recommended thru the vet as she or he might in all likelihood want to regulate their meal plans in step with any precise concerns or illnesses currently worrying your domestic dog.

An computerized meals dispenser may be your extremely good pal (apart from your hairy accomplice) if you spend extended hours at paintings each day. Even in case you feed your canine as fast as you get again domestic, it's high-quality to time table timed feedings in your doggy, especially considering puppies surely thrive on everyday.

Many canine feeders can be timed to adjust your pup's consuming time table, and you get to pick how an awful lot you need to feed on a day by day foundation, as nicely. This may additionally even assist if your canine has a bent to wake you up early inside the morning, annoying to be fed.

Feeders can artwork with wet or dry meals relying on the model, and excellent manufacturers cater to excellent sizes.

Timed 12-meal automatic feeders are taken into consideration the notable and healthiest alternative for small or medium-sized dogs. This manner, in preference to ingesting massive food, they're fed 12 smaller meals at some level inside the day. The gradual feed mode slowly dispenses meals over the path of 15 mins to prevent your canine from vomiting, which usually takes place even as puppies devour too speedy.

But that doesn't advocate that the gadget receives to select whilst and the way your canine eats. If you need to set an ingesting schedule to your dog for your private terms for scientific motives, there's a right away feed mode that lets in you to choose the a part of food served as properly.

For big dogs, five-meal feeders may be set to serve more generous portions, and some component time desk you select out out automatically rotates to day after today. Unlike its 12-meal counterpart, this dispenser works super with dry further to moist food.

Whatever dispenser you pick out in your dog, ensure you are taking out the tray or bowl to clean it each day.

Dog house

Dogs want to usually be allowed to return again inner each time they need to, however in the event that they regularly spend time for your out of doors (and that they probably will), it's outstanding to install a comfortable dog house for them.

For starters, this creates a region for them that they feel is their own. Just like your own family members have a room of their private, a dog house might be your domestic dog's private place. Dog houses can also protect your pets from warmth strokes; but, if it's even fairly heat for you outdoor, it's probable too warm on your dog. Make sure that some thing canine door you've got installed can be locked at the same time as necessary, so that you can keep your buddy interior whilst the weather situations are not best.

You don't need to spend hundreds of dollars on custom-made dog houses that healthy the out of doors layout of your own home. Any commonplace den made of white cedar is probably pretty durable, and moreover secure for your canine. White cedar is also referred to as stained white timber, and the motive why it makes the proper cloth for dog houses is that it's genuinely non-poisonous for pets and offers off a pleasant fragrance although wet.

Aside from being an aesthetically attractive addition in your outside, it's additionally resistant to extreme weather changes further to pests which could infest your lawn, so you can relaxation assured that your canine may be constant underneath its little sloped roof.

If you're going to make your purchase on-line, make certain you choose the right duration. If you advise on adopting a domestic canine, larger sizes are needless. Dogs, in enormous, enjoy at ease areas, so some thing too commodious on your fur toddler isn't always recommended. Whatever you pick out out, we recommend you get one with floor panels, so your canine doesn't need to take a sleep on a wet garden.

Grooming package deal

You need to as a minimum have a number one grooming package at domestic, even if you plan to regularly take your dog to a professional groomer.

Grooming isn't pretty a great deal preserving your dog looking adorable. Trimming a dog's fur and nails frequently is sanitary and permits you spot any signs of capability infections or illnesses. Grooming your pup often may also additionally even lower coat and pores and pores and skin troubles like everyday scratching, rashes, bumps, and matting. Combing your canine's hair lightly distributes hair oils, because of this your dog will have a extra healthy and shinier coat.

Grooming is also healthier for the dog's human companion as it cuts down on allergens like shed hair.

Your package must normally have a comb, scissors, trimmers, and clippers. Depending at the breed, many dogs can be specially afraid of loud clippers. There are many silent ones within the marketplace in particular created for timid puppies. If you're unsure if your dog will take grooming well, pass for the silent package, and recollect that its belief of this revel in can generally be stepped forward with masses of love, reward, and treats.

Before grooming, make sure your canine is bathed. If your dog regularly plays out of doors, a weekly tub must suffice. Do not shower your dog extra than as speedy as weekly.

If your own home canine has a thick coat, untangle any knots earlier than you shower it. Use lukewarm water and diluted canine shampoo. Never use cleaning soap or human shampoo on puppies, irrespective of the truth that some humans also can choose to use horse shampoo for thicker and shinier coats.

With effective breeds, you'll want to spend money on a stripping knife. Dogs that do not surely shed hair will need you to manually strip overgrown and useless hair. Make sure your dog is comfortable with being stripped, in any other case this procedure can be extremely inconvenient for every you and your pup.

Use nail clippers to hold your dog's nails trimmed. If you don't reduce them often, they'll be extra difficult to reduce the following time you attempt to do it. Standard scissors artwork awesome, however we advocate the guillotine clipper. If you bypass this step, it becomes more and more difficult on your canine to walk, as their nails will develop into a curve that pricks at their paws as they waft spherical.

Aside from trimming nails and hair, ensure you regularly comb your dog to remove any shed hair and preserve its coat easy and tangle-free.

Collars and leashes

Although they will be the most apparent ones at the listing, they're genuinely crucial gadgets no matter in that you're preserving your home dog till it grows up. Walking your domestic dog can assist the two of you bond, and will make it turn out to be more comfortable round people.

When it includes collars, ID tags are critical to make sure that your puppy will usually be diagnosed in case it loses its manner. Puppies are commonly hyperactive and amusing-loving, so ensure that your leash is a great healthful; in any other case, you may lose your grip in case your doggy sees a familiar neighbor inside the distance, or a stray animal it wants to chase.

No rely what type of leash or collar you get your canine, no matter the reality that, now not a few thing might be as stable as getting it microchipped, so that you can allow you to discover precisely in which it's miles. If a microchipped dog ever receives out of place and a person takes it to a vet, they may use your records to touch you and produce your dog once more.

When deciding on collars, ensure it's the right in form. Collars which are too tight may be fantastically uncomfortable to your dog, at the same time as others can also additionally additionally slip off with out problem. Whatever you choose, make certain which you have extras lying around so you can without difficulty replace them inside the occasion that they wander off.

Carrier

Carriers for larger puppies are complex commercial company, however it's no longer a few aspect that your nearby pet store cannot guide you thru. Your puppy will probable in shape in any plastic carrier, but as your dog grows up, you'll discover your self switching amongst bigger sizes.

You need to usually realize the load and measurements of your canine in advance than you head to a puppy store. Measure your dog from the lowest of its neck to the inspiration of its tail, then add a few inches for the top and tail. The pinnacle must moreover be calculated, and the load of your canine contributes to the material you'll choose to make certain it's strong enough in your canine's period.

There are plastic and timber corporations, further to mild-sided ones. It all relies upon on how you plan to apply them. If you're to your way to a flight, mild-sided vendors can with out problems be located under seats. But if your canine is travelling in cargo, ensure the organization is tough, robust, and most significantly, nicely-ventilated.

If you're using your provider for vet trips, backpack agencies paintings brilliant for smaller puppies. Bigger puppies can easily be carried to a vehicle or taken on public transportation.

Whatever provider you purchase, ensure it is long lasting. If you cheap out for your pet shopping spree, you'll probable grow to be repurchasing the whole thing. Bear in mind that puppies can without issues get away reasonably-priced material vendors.

Dog mattress

It doesn't rely in case you plan to have your dog sleep next to you; your doggy need to constantly have a mattress of its very private. Just like canine houses, canine beds are part of your excellent pal's private bubble. And the truth is, dogs will in all likelihood select their very very personal beds over yours.

There are masses of dog beds on hand, and each is primarily based upon at the drowsing style of your canine. You can get a sprawler, a burrower, a roller, or a leaner. Shape and layout apart, you want to make sure that you buy the right period, which isn't too spacious or too small on your dog.

You'll locate exquisite material in the marketplace. Most of them don't make a difference, as long as you test the label or description of the product and ensure that it's machine-washer-friendly, bearing in mind that dog beds will want to be washed often.

Piddle pads and newspapers

Unfortunately, a few dogs may be hard to teach, and the number one few weeks at your property will probably be a chunk of a nightmare. Adding to that is the fact that puppies have a tendency to leak, so you'll need to preserve your private home stocked with all forms of education pads and line the flooring with newspapers till your doggy gets the lay of the land. While you're at it, you'll probable need to cover your couches and beds in vinyl due to the fact opportunities are, your new package deal deal of cuteness will involuntarily wet them, so it's first-class to err at the component of caution.

A veterinarian

While that's no longer some factor you could get at the shop, it's a few factor you need to be prepared for earlier than you adopt a trendy domestic dog.

Some human beings have a tendency to endure in thoughts vet centers as places your pet most effective wishes to go to whilst it's ill. But the fact is, you're going to need to invest in monthly visits for ordinary check-ups. Even in case your canine is acting the identical, there's a ton of clinical complications that may be detected thru your vet, ideally at early degrees.

There also are times whilst your dog can also appear okay, however is in reality enduring an ache, allergies, or a developing infection.

That stated, your dog will must be regularly dewormed and will in the long run need to be neutered or spayed, if this hasn't already been finished with the useful aid of the safe haven. Ask the rescuer of your puppy if it has already been vaccinated so your vet is privy to what he/she is managing.

Don't absolutely pick out the closest vet to your house. Make powerful you take a look at evaluations earlier than you make a decision to do not forget a vet with your home canine. If taking your dog to the vet is an excessive amount of of a hassle, home visits are also an alternative, but can be quite more expensive.

Even in spite of the reality that getting a canine may sound like a heartwarming concept, it's furthermore a large responsibility. So, earlier than you're making the huge choice, ensure that your art work time table lets in you to put money into mentioning a doggy. And if this is the primary puppy you personal, ensure to touch your community vet earlier than you convey your dog home, to be made aware about the test-u.S.You'll want to make to keep your canine happy and healthy.

Chapter 2: A Happy Home

Now that you've made the large preference and organized your house or apartment in your new fur infant, the subsequent step is to make certain it receives aware about its environment as quick as feasible, and makes itself at domestic! In order to advantage this, you'll want to decide on a few key factors concerning its weight loss program and normal, and form a tremendous bond collectively along with your home canine. In time, each of you could get a better facts of approaches subjects may be running spherical your vicinity, however for now, you can start via using focusing in your dog's nutrients and its way of speakme with you, so as not to miss any critical symptoms it is probably imparting you with regarding its happiness and nicely-being.

How and When to Feed Your Puppy

Once you've got were given a satisfied little pooch constantly presenting you with the house dog eyes for the following mealtime, you'll understand how crucial it is which you understand what it need to be ingesting, and the way often you must feed it. So, proper right here's a feeding guide that will help you wrap your head round it.

What ought to you feed your domestic dog?

When it includes organisation meals, you'll discover canned or semi-moist meals, or kibble. When identifying which one your pup must be ingesting, it's far exquisite to no longer best understand what it modified into formerly feeding on, but additionally what the vet recommends for its nutritional necessities. It is certainly really worth noting that kibble is generally the most inside your finances and realistic preference, but a few dogs are vulnerable to be allergic to a number of the components. If you're changing from one type to every different, it's miles first-rate to make the trade progressively, so it's smooth at the doggy's belly and doesn't bring about digestion problems.

Wet food vs dry food

The trap 22 state of affairs of whether or not or no longer to choose moist or dry meals is actual. But, in case you need to make a calculated choice, you need to first recognize why every one is important on your puppy. It is properly surely well worth bringing up that counting on the proper emblem of dog meals you'll be buying, the additives and nutrients it consists of, further to its consistency may also variety dramatically. That said, every type does include a few benefits.

Wet meals

While moist food is normally greater high priced, it can be extra beneficial for your dog. You'll be aware that moist food is more immoderate in odor as it has a more potent flavor, making it preferred through dogs to dry meals in the event that they had been given a desire. Another essential difference is that on account that moist meals has plenty greater liquid in it, it is able to make up for a number of your dog's required water intake. So, in case your canine has problem eating water, then it's far endorsed to feed it moist food—regardless of the truth that dehydration is a first-rate trouble in puppies, so don't depend in fact at the moisture content material fabric of canned food. For dogs that will be inclined to overeat and turn out to be overweight, wet food may also be a higher alternative as it has a decrease quantity of energy content cloth material, which permits them to eat more without exceeding their calorie consumption.

If kibble isn't always in fact your problem but the price of buying wet food for the rest of your canine's life additionally appears a chunk overwhelming, you can moreover prepare sparkling, home made meals on your hairy pal. In that case, you could feed it a uncooked diet plan, which has many demonstrated fitness blessings, or perform a bit research to discover some balanced, home-cooked dog meals recipes on-line. Dry food

You'll find out that the commonplace form of kibble has a tendency to be much less pricey than moist meals. You'll furthermore find out a full-size type of options to help you pick out the splendid on your dog. Another component to go through in mind is that thinking about that dry food is actually dry, it doesn't flow into terrible as fast as moist food and may be overlooked on the same time as you're at paintings or travelling with out you having to fear. Dry food also generally contains a higher quantity of strength assets, because of this a smaller amount is wanted an awesome manner to satisfy the canine's day by day food consumption requirements. You'll word that dry food typically has a miles plenty less wonderful heady scent, making it greater accessible to miss without the entire house smelling like dog food. However, when you have a picky eater, you would likely should decorate the scent and taste through the use of the use of which incorporates some hen broth or a few "toppers" to its food.

When it includes dry food, you'll find some of alternatives with a vast kind of costs. While you might be tempted to move for the most inexpensive desire, bear in mind the reality that the rate varies consistent with the extraordinary of the components. So, with a view to ensure that your home canine is getting the nutrients it dreams, it's miles amazing to pick out as a minimum a mid-variety emblem to assure that it gets the desired vitamins without spending too much coins. No rely which kind of food or brand making a decision on, don't neglect to carefully observe the labels, and higher however, go to your vet.

What vitamins are important for your home canine?

Always double-check the elements to make certain that they're rich in protein as a way to assist assist your domestic dog's muscle groups and boom. It is also vital to have carbohydrates blanketed inside the eating regimen, as it materials the domestic dog with the electricity had to play and be lively. Calcium is some other essential detail because it helps the improvement of teeth and bones, mainly while a whelp remains growing, and omega-3 fatty acids are crucial a great way to maintain a healthful brain, heart, kidney, and coat, in addition to strengthening the immune system.

How regularly need to you feed your pup?

Depending on the scale and age of your furball, the feeding agenda will range.

6-12 weeks

During this time, a home canine needs to be feeding extra frequently so one can make sure growth and that's why it's far wonderful to feed it around four instances in keeping with day. However, it's far critical to pick out meals that the pup's stomach can digest, so you need to choose out a type of canine meals that's specifically designed for dogs.

three-6 months

Once your home dog has grown and has started out developing, it is time to lower the kind of times it eats and bring it down to a few times an afternoon alternatively.

6-one year

If you've determined your domestic canine is developing healthily into a hint doggie, then it is recommended to pleasant feed it times a day. You can provide one portion of dog meals earlier than you go away the residence within the morning and pinnacle off for a 2nd serving after you get lower lower again. This want to be enough meals in your dog, but you'll have the ability to inform with the useful resource of the usage of the constant whimpering if it gets hungry greater often and is in want of a better dosage. During this period, it's also endorsed to replace from domestic canine to character meals, at round eight months when you have a small breed. However, if you have a bigger breed, then it's miles great to wait till it turns thirteen months to replace to man or woman food.

When it includes vitamins, it is constantly critical to get a session from your vet to help you determine what sort of food your canine not simplest needs, but will experience the most. It might also moreover take a few trial and mistakes inside the starting, however don't fear—so long as a manner to look for all of the signs and symptoms, your doggy will can help you recognise whether or not or no longer its contemporary diet plan appears to be strolling for it or now not.

Stress Signals You Should Look Out For

For many people, it takes some time to get used to napping in a bed that isn't their own. So, recollect how a home canine need to experience at the equal time as it's not most effective modified the vicinity, however the complete surroundings, such as owners—doesn't that sound worrying? That's why it is essential to preserve a watch out for any of those symptoms and signs and symptoms to determine if your new member of the family desires a few greater care and soothing.

Body Language

A domestic is a dog's safe sanctuary and moving to a brand new domestic might be causing your little pup a whole lot of tension, particularly on the identical time as it's unexpected with you and doesn't apprehend how stable it need to be feeling round you. One of the maximum common symptoms and signs and symptoms and signs to suggest that your domestic dog is feeling burdened may be via its frame language. Shaking and shivering are apparent signs of pain and worry, similarly to annoying muscle companies and immoderate drooling. If your doggy is itching and scratching plenty, or dropping more hair than it need to be, those are all signs and symptoms and signs and symptoms that will help you recognize that it's forced.

Position of ears

While it might be difficult to test because you're uncommon with the normal feature of your new home dog's ears, maximum puppies generally generally tend to both perk up their ears once they're in a demanding state of affairs or pull their ears again in opposition to their heads.

Eyes

Dogs' eyes, much like humans', can show masses approximately how they're feeling. When a pup is feeling confused or going via a frightening state of affairs, it commonly gives you the issue-eye with a white crescent shape appearing around its eyes. This 1/2 of-moon eye is a common sign that your terrible doggy is freaking out and is in want of soothing.

Barking

While it's far normal for puppies to bark, barking for no purpose may be a robust indication of strain—mainly after they no longer handiest bark, but additionally inn to whimpering, whining, growling and immoderate panting. This may be because of separation tension from its mom or previous proprietor, or signs and symptoms and signs of stress at the way to get up until it feels extra snug and greater secure round you.

Destroying residence device

Because your puppy is uncommon with the surroundings, it could lodge to destroying fixtures, doorways, or a few aspect it can get its arms on—or paws in this example. While it's miles a everyday reaction to get mad, it's far important to apprehend that this is only due to the stress of being in an surprising environment and could want time to settle in.

There are many signs and signs and symptoms that your pup is feeling harassed, but it's far important to recognize that this isn't always handiest commonplace, however furthermore very legitimate for it to experience this way. This is the time whilst the house canine wants to feel that it's miles part of a modern-day family a terrific way to manual it and smother it with love. It is remarkable to preserve your house canine close, pup it if viable, deliver it food and water to expose which you care, while trying to installation a connection to make the stress and anxiety leave.

Taking care of a domestic dog isn't commonly an clean task, but so long as you're prepared, invested and retaining a be cautious for what your maximum current family member desires, you'll be doing a exceptional hobby. Sure, giving your buddy the great dog food you can come up with the cash for will be very critical, but at the give up of the day, canine possession includes masses more than supplying food, water, and shelter. Remember that from the instant your home canine walks thru the door, your house might be its home, too. Ensuring that it's a happy one will take some time and try, however it'll sincerely be worth it.

Chapter 3: Training Your Puppy

Training can be very essential in a dog's life. It creates a stronger bond some of the doggy and the proprietor, and performs into the dog's splendid of existence through imparting it with the important highbrow stimulation. It permits the canine installation right from wrong using rewards for suitable conduct, and correction for terrible conduct. Dogs need these precious education to enjoy solid, consistent, assured and satisfied. Training need to not involve hurtful behavior, and correction have to in no way include any form of abuse. It's important which you in no manner use shaming techniques in case your canine isn't pretty getting the draw close of it however; it's going to take time and getting annoyed gained't assist. Training is ready encouraging your canine to behave in strategies which can be great in your own home and in public places.

Basic education

You can begin simple schooling collectively together with your domestic dog from to 4 months antique. Start with easy commands consisting of "take a seat down" earlier than you supply it a meal. Be affected individual collectively with your dog, and reward its compliance with treats. Gradually flow directly to "come" and "stay." Don't spend extra than ten minutes a day on tricks, and don't confuse it thru education 5 commands proper now.

Will you need to lease a teacher?

Hiring a trainer is usually recommended for first-time canine proprietors as the amount of schooling data handy can be overwhelming. However, even when you have masses of experience raising canine companions, you can commonly enhance your competencies with training experts. Obedience faculties are highly advocated as they no longer nice teach your dog number one to superior schooling, however moreover they beautify your canine's social competencies—it honestly is of top notch significance—in addition to offer you with the gear to keep its development.

How will you recognize which instructor is right for you?

Ask questions. Find out what the instructor's philosophy is based on what strategies they use. It's pleasant to choose training colleges that use exquisite reinforcement for appropriate behavior, coaching possibility behaviors to put in vicinity of beside the point ones. It's vital you experience snug with them, and consider them collectively together with your pup.

What to assume

Change takes time as dogs study thru repetition and choose up instructions step by step. Like children, your puppy will go through a difficult phase as it checks its barriers. Do no longer come to be annoyed; this is normal and as long as you live calm and preserve training as a quick and fun enjoy, they'll hop decrease lower back on board.

Training want to continuously be a laugh and embody masses of praise. Your dog want to develop familiar with the phrase "best female/boy" and understand that it's encouragement. This way, it will possibly be happier, and your bond may be stronger while it's given easy obstacles.

Getting Your Puppy's Focus

At one thing or a few different, you want to face the challenge of training your canine. This can be alternatively difficult at the start, but the extra you workout, the higher and less hard it receives. One rule of thumb, even though, is to capture your pup's hobby and keep it focused. There are many straightforward and amusing bodily video video games to do assist you do in truth that, and proper here are a number of them.

The eye touch exercise

Eye touch is one of the most critical subjects that your home dog desires to research. It teaches your little pooch a way to sit down

down quietly, genuinely dedicating its interest to you. All you want to do is get a few treats and take a seat beside your domestic dog. When your presence grabs its hobby, reward it with some treats. Be affected person as you strive out this workout and repeat it extra than as fast as to make sure that your puppy becomes aware about the relationship.

The hand targeted on exercise

Hand focused on training is understood to be one of the empowering sports in your dog. It is quite easy to do. All you need to do is place the palm of your hand in the the front of your domestic dog's nostril. Once your little domestic dog touches your hand, reward it with some treats and repeat it time and again again. This exercising especially lets in your puppy stay targeted and forget approximately about each different distractions that is probably round.

The impulse control exercising

This exercising is extra or lots much less a concept that has many versions for you and your home canine to work with. You usually begin this after you make sure that your home dog is well-knowledgeable in keeping eye contact. To train your domestic dog impulse manipulate, strive losing some element from the table to the floor. If your doggy rushes to get it, cover it together together with your foot as your dog strategies. If it patiently sits and waits, reward your home canine with its very very own treats. If it attempts to achieve the food, location your foot lower decrease lower back at the meals and repeat.

The distraction exercising

Distraction is what specifically affects your puppy's cognizance and interest. For this kind of exercise, you will be desiring topics: a quiet place to exercising, and a clicker or a toy that your domestic dog responds to.

Once you're ready, you could start education your dog the manner to reputation on a few thing precise with the resource of the usage of the sound of the clicker or its favored toy. Either of those gadgets will grasp its attention and assist it focus. After you've practiced for a while, you may start to steadily boom the quantity of distractions around for higher outcomes.

Being affected character is an important factor of education your domestic canine. Not without a doubt everybody are education specialists in fact. However, the extra you figure on those sporting occasions together with your puppy, the sooner it's going to discover ways to be privy to its education classes.

Teaching Your Puppy Its Name

This may moreover sound easy enough; all you want to do is deliver your puppy a name, use it regularly, and that's it. Sooner or later your doggy will get used to it, proper? While this can be right, there's extra you could do to train your home canine its call in a manner that permits you to apply it as a device to possibly keep it secure.

By calling your canine's call whilst it's approximately to wander into hazard, you could prevent many capability failures, however most effective if the dog absolutely turns once more to you on every occasion. With this in thoughts, permit's check the way to teach your pup its call in a extra hooked up manner.

Get your doggy's interest

Start this way whilst you're at domestic with out a distractions spherical and a deliver of treats to apply a reward. Make high excellent which you have already got your canine's hobby earlier than you start, and keep away from schooling if your canine is tired, overexcited, or distracted. Call your canine's call in a warmness, pleased tone and straight away reward it with a treat at the same time as it appears at you.

In most instances, your home dog will examine you in reality to see what's occurring, however the incentive of getting a treat will permit it to associate its call with some element brilliant and encourage it to look again the subsequent time you name its name.

Now, allow your puppy's interest wander and then name its name once more. As quickly because it appears at you, reward it yet again with a treat. Repeat those steps for a maximum of 10 times in a single consultation and preserve the education quick. If you overdo it, your domestic canine will become bored and lose interest, rendering the whole approach useless.

Change the education vicinity

Start mixing up the locations in which you've got your training lessons, however stay indoors. Choose locations with minimal distractions because of the truth you're nevertheless early on inside the schooling manner and you want to set your property dog as lots as win. Repeat the previous steps round your house and outdoor in masses of training inside the path of the day till you could successfully get your puppy's hobby every time.

Increase the time you require its interest

Now, you have to attempt to growth the time you require its interest earlier than worthwhile it. Call your domestic dog's name and on the same time as it gives you its hobby, praise it immediately, but appearance beforehand to multiple seconds in advance than giving it the cope with. This way, you educate it to offer you its interest for longer. Gradually increase the time until you could subsequently keep your pup's undivided hobby for as a minimum 5 seconds every time you name it.

Introduce distractions

Once you may reliably count on maintaining your doggy's interest for at least 5 seconds in a controlled environment, growth the problem diploma of the education with the useful resource of introducing a few distractions. Have a person else be present inside the room, deliver the canine a toy, or perhaps even turn the TV on. Wait until it's in reality distracted, then name its name. Because this is extra tough than the preceding wearing activities, praise your doggy proper now even as it appears at you rather than searching in advance to five seconds.

Move it outdoor

Now that you could get your puppy's hobby indoors even though distracted, it's time to take it up a notch and flow into your education outdoor. Start somewhere quiet and flow lower again to the simple wearing activities that require a limited hobby span, then step by step artwork your manner inside the path of the more tough bodily video video games.

This might also moreover seem like loads of paintings clearly to teach your puppy its call, however that's first-class because of the reality you're going to use it as an effective device in numerous situations. Whether it's for purchasing your home dog's hobby in any scenario, ensuring its protection, or education it extra effectively, the ones hints assist you to effectively gather all that with the least strive possible.

What Is a Clicker Word and Why Is It Important?

There are lots of factors that you need to study as a new dog owner, and an entire lot of education to do. Every canine owner is aware of that they want to start training their dogs as early as viable. People begin with clean things like schooling their canine its name, until it steadily reaches a snug degree where it is able to apprehend the clicker signal.

What is a clicker phrase?

The clicker itself is a drastically small system this is used to talk together together with your puppy. This device has a small button that releases a noise even as clicked on and lets your canine understand that it'll probable be getting a address for a system nicely completed. However, you don't always want to use that tool. You can use a clicker word of your deciding on; it may be anything you need. It additionally can be a brilliant sound like a clap or a whistle. If your dog is deaf, you may talk by using the use of using the usage of slight. The crucial trouble is to have a clicker word or a sign, some thing it could be.

Shaping the canine's behavior

Puppies need to be right now professional as quickly as they may be in your property, and this is in which the clicker word comes into play. One of the first topics you may be teaching your dog is potty schooling. The clicker word can be helping you with this. You will need to take have a look at of your canine's conduct, and praise it whenever it does its enterprise out of doors in place of internal. You say the clicker phrase as fast as it's miles finished after which offer it a address. You can exercise this technique with the whole thing else which you need your canine to do.

Communication

Unfortunately, humans and puppies don't have a everyday language they may be capable of use to talk. This is precisely why your home dog desires to look at some matters, beginning with its name. Let's say you want to call out on your canine as it's lunchtime; how are you going to try this without using its call? The clicker allows you with that, too. Start with the resource of grabbing the canine's hobby, call out its name, and on the identical time because it responds, say the clicker word and then supply it a treat. Do this repetitively, till you call out for it and it comes to you proper away. This manner, your canine friends its call with a deal with and is aware about that it did an notable hobby with the aid of manner of the usage of responding, due to the reality you said the clicker word.

You may have discovered that the clicker word and treats circulate hand-in-hand. But this is only within the beginning. You want to set up that the clicker word way "you likely did a high-quality interest." So, you may first rate be the usage of the treats at the start at the identical time as the dog continues to be greater youthful. Later on, you could find yourself the use of the clicker phrase without having accessible out treats. Dogs are sensible beings, so don't worry; the getting to know method gained't take extended.

Teaching Your Dog to Recognize and Listen to Your Voice

Getting your puppy to be privy to you and examine your instructions isn't always any easy project, and it simplest comes from an area of take delivery of as actual with and affection. That is why that is the great location to start while you get your new fur toddler. After years of trial and errors, humans have decided some essential guidelines to govern your canine's behaviors and make it observe your instructions, be they sounds, gestures, or perhaps a glance.

First and most vital, be the boss

Dogs admire authority. Show your domestic dog who's the leader from day one. Start through continuously walking one step in advance and status over it while giving a command. Make positive it's miles familiar with that you may now not tolerate unaccepted behavior. Using a agency tone of voice—this isn't always just like a median one, and in reality no longer shouting—while giving commands will lay down the floor tips about who is to be observed in this courting.

Lead with the aid of encouragement

Reward your dog to lure it into paying attention to you. You can start by using using presenting treats on every occasion it follows an order. If it responds to its name, make certain you deliver that that is the desired conduct and praise it no matter most effective a pat at the lower returned and an encouraging "appropriate boy." Once you have a look at that your dog has determined out this trick and it's now not new to it, bypass on and keep the treats for the subsequent lesson. Refrain from upsetting your pup into submission through irritated demeanor, as this will high-quality make it mistrust you and function a horrible impact in your relationship.

Consistency is essential

Just like people, being sent combined messages confuses puppies. Common phrases and movements are for use with all people of the own family and some other character to deal with your property canine. Actions like "sit down down," "live" or "roll" want to be unified with the proper same wording continually.

Make time for training

Dedicate a part of your every day recurring for domestic dog schooling. Think of it as your excellent time along with your domestic dog.

Go for walks or play a couple of minutes of fetch before beginning your session. This way, your pup can get beyond its excitement and launch stored power to have a mainly easy mind and cognizance to your education. Experts recommend schooling in 15-minute instructions every day, repeating every command five-15 times earlier than shifting immediately to the subsequent one.

Affirm your instructions visually

Assigning an movement to each voice order makes the gaining knowledge of device easier for puppies. Demanding your dog to sit may be discovered thru manner of shifting the palm of your hand going thru downwards in repetition. This manner, your canine can be tuned to every your voice and body gestures. This technique is specifically useful for dogs with taking note of troubles, or senior ones.

Practice in specific setups

Puppies can behave perfectly at home, then get honestly distracted at the same time as it's playtime in the park. If you keep working towards in unique environments, your dog will recognize that irrespective of in which you're, a command is a command and desires to be accompanied. As prolonged as it's miles a stable region, display your dog which you assume obedience anywhere.

Consider expert advice

Seek guidance from specialists to assist with conduct alternate and help your canine examine faster. You can get keep of recommendation on the way to brilliant skip approximately the schooling. However, don't forget to ask for references from different canine mother and father beforehand. You also can watch movement photographs and attend workshops designed to suit your precise desires.

Do not surrender

Keep repeating your practices again and again yet again. The time it takes to finish the education of laying command varies from one dog to the possibility. Study the tendencies of your doggy's breed and do the vital studies to control your expectancies and avoid being pissed off; otherwise, you will be putting in place your dog for failure as it selections up for your energy and vibe.

Dogs are sincerely guy's best pals, and that they'll sincerely do their awesome to delight their owners once they get the draw close of things. It may additionally take your canine some time to apprehend what you're in reality asking, but be affected character and attempt to take this technique one step at a time. Once you every get used to every exclusive and shape a tremendous records, the love and happiness it brings into your life will virtually be properly well worth the attempt you positioned into its training.

Basic Commands All Puppies Should Learn

It is without a doubt a laugh to look at a dog roll over and play vain on command, however allow's admit it; the ones are a piece too advanced in your new domestic dog to carry out just however. Training has a sure shape and not unusual enjoy to it, and it makes yours—and your dog's—existence much less complex in case you stick to toddler steps. There are sure commands which may be less complex to understand than others for max dogs, and they may be able to are available in reality reachable in ordinary lifestyles, even contributing in your fur toddler's safety and protection in a few conditions. Here are some easy commands that every doggy ought to study inside the early levels of the education approach.

Sit

You'll discover that maximum professionals agree that the "take a seat down" command is the very first-class for puppies to have a look at, and it's moreover one of the maximum important ones. This is why it is also the number one one they're taught. It teaches them undertaking, and primarily based mostly on that, they start responding to simple training. To train your property dog the "sit down down" command, you want to be slight and top notch, worthwhile it with treats and reward each time it gets it right. You in truth need to keep a deal with for your hand, after which located it near your dog's nose so it might recognize what it's miles. It could probable most probable try to reach up and get it, that is even as you need to lightly guide it down along with your distinct hand on the identical time as saying "take a seat." When it follows your command, doggy it and offer it the cope with. You can also appoint mealtimes by using the usage of defensive the food bowl up on your hand and looking on your dog to sit naturally with the resource of manner of itself, then worthwhile it with the food once it does. Keep repeating the ones techniques till your domestic dog instinctively responds to the command upon listening to it as quickly as.

Some dogs don't respond properly to being touched or manually handled inside the path of training. In that case, you can hold a deal with to your hand above your dog's head whilst it's miles status within the front of a wall or an object, and circulate your hand in the route of its again at the same time as saying "sit." It will maximum probable take a seat down by using itself as a manner to attention at the address without being able to glide again. When it does, say the clicker word and supply the address.

Down

This is a comparable command to "take a seat" and it's particularly beneficial with big puppies, as it makes them lie down in a comfortable function. When they get used to mendacity down on command, it turns into much less hard to take them out to parks and consuming locations, because they'd be exciting on the ground with out you having to fear about them all the time. You can teach your canine this smooth command pretty resultseasily similar to the previous one, but you'll located the address a piece further proper right down to the ground this time and pretty in the direction of you. You'll find out that the canine is following you down and stretching beforehand in the direction of the cope with. Keep announcing the command, and even as its belly touches the ground, say the clicker word and deliver it the deal with. Repeat each day until it has it memorized.

If your dog has a tendency to comply with the address without touching the floor, you can limit its region with the useful resource of the use of your very own legs. Sit down on the ground along with your decrease once more leaning in opposition to a wall and bend your knees to form a form of 'tunnel' alongside aspect your legs. Make your dog follow the treat on your hand, defensive it at the opportunity problem of your legs. While trying to find to benefit the cope with, it'll likely have to flow into below your bent legs, being compelled to move slowly on the ground. Once it reaches this function and touches the ground with its entire body, say the clicker phrase and praise your dog.

Heel

The "heel" command is one of the most important ones to be had, because it teaches your domestic dog to walk next to you instead of direction lower lower back or try to outrun you. It teaches dogs location and the way to stroll subsequent to their owners without inflicting any issues. It additionally allows them to get used to being walked on a leash. This one might be a piece trickier to teach, but with some exercise, your pooch receives there. You can use a squeaky toy for this one, and also you begin via putting a collar and a leash at the house canine. Then you order it to take a seat down, and ask it to observe from that function with the squeaky toy on your hand as you start moving forward. As you stroll, repeat the command "heel," and if the home canine receives distracted, use the toy to make it popularity. If it tries to outrun you, pause and supply it the toy and reward it for pausing with you. After it's extra focused, attempt repeating all over again until it can examine up with you with out lagging within the lower back of or looking to outrun you.

Come

A lot of humans consider the "come" command to be the maximum important of they all, due to the fact it'd simply grow to be saving your existence or that of your canine ultimately. Puppies need to be trained this one early on, and you want to be diligent with it, as they want to truly recognize a way to look at this command. It might likely show up inside the destiny that your dog escapes its leash or runs in the course of a capability risk. This command can maintain it from being hit by way of a automobile or drawing near strangers. So, it has so that you can proper now run once more to you as quick as it hears the phrase. You need to by no means scold your canine if it fails to collect this even as known as, and be very affected character—it'd get the wrong message and in reality keep away from you if this results in trauma. Use its preferred toy or deal with to trap it at the same time as repeating the command, and be very beneficiant with praise on the same time as it does come inside the course of you. It's a reasonably easy order to teach, but it can take the time until your doggy can get used to it, and also you shouldn't rush it the least bit.

Leave it / don't contact

Dogs are curious creatures through nature, and that interest can get them in trouble pretty regularly. This is in which the "depart it" command comes in; it can defend them from drawing close to a doubtlessly risky item. It also facilitates during the house if your domestic dog is gambling with some thing it ought to live far from. This command is a bit complex to educate dogs, so you need to be affected man or woman with this one as properly. You can method it thru retaining treats in every arms, and even as the doggy tries to approach one, repeat the command "go away it." When it does, offer it the deal with in the wonderful hand, and praise it. That manner, your canine will begin getting used to the concept that some subjects are off-limits, and so long as you preserve repeating the word and profitable it, it'll be quite responsive even as you order it to move away a few thing.

The critical trouble is to be affected man or woman and effective with a number of those instructions. Puppies need steady motivation and pampering so as to respond to training, and that they do need to get pampered. So, take some time even as training them new topics, and produce a number of toys and treats! Nothing locations a puppy within the temper to cooperate like treats and being referred to as an extraordinary doggie.

How to Housebreak Your Puppy

Housebreaking is vital for a happy courting between a domestic canine proprietor and their domestic dog. In order to potty teach your home canine, you'll should research a few matters your self. Below are a few attempted-and-examined training recommendations that will help you successfully residence-train your domestic canine.

When should you begin?

One of the most vital steps you want to take for a satisfied existence collectively with your pup is coaching it to relieve itself on the right time and place. Dog professionals recommend that you start potty education your domestic canine while it's round three months vintage because via that age it's going to have sufficient bladder and bowel manage to discover ways to maintain it.

How prolonged does it take?

It normally takes 4 to six months for a domestic dog to be clearly potty skilled, however, the length can variety appreciably from one puppy to every different; a few can be fast beginners while others can absorb to a twelve months. This relies upon on many elements at the side of the canine's age, man or woman, previous residing situations, and breed. For instance, smaller puppies along side pugs and chihuahuas have smaller bladders and better metabolisms, because of this that that they've to go more frequently.

And the more your doggy has to transport, the extra you want to educate it.

Basic housebreaking foundations

Besides the commonplace walks out of doors, there are primary approaches to potty schooling your domestic dog; crate education and paper training. Each method has its execs and cons but they might all paintings if you observe the critical regulations of burglary. Regardless of the education method you choose, professionals recommend confining the domestic canine to a selected space or room until it learns to do its company inside the proper vicinity. Then, you can frequently deliver it extra freedom to roam about the house.

Routine

If you fail to be steady, your domestic canine will fail, too. So, make sure to maintain a consistent time table to your doggy. This consists of its journeys outdoor, feeding times, and exercise physical games. Stick to a regular feeding schedule on your doggie and do away with its food amongst food; this way, you could modify the times even as it'll need to alleviate itself. When taking your doggy outside, supply it to the equal spot each time due to the fact its heady scent will prompt it to do its organization there.

Encouragement

If your doggy gets it proper, reward it with treats, praise, or affection to enhance its real conduct. But if it does some aspect wrong, make it clean which you're no longer glad with it by means of ignoring it or firmly announcing "no." Whatever you do, don't hit your puppy, due to the fact this teaches it to fear you in vicinity of love you, and this can not make it observe any quicker. In truth, it'll probable expand the whole training manner.

Correction

If you seize your dog within the act, say "no" in a sharp tone or clap loudly so it'd understand that it's performing some aspect wrong. When it stops, take it to its particular spot to complete its industrial corporation, and then reward it or deliver it a small deal with at the same time as it's carried out. Thoroughly easy up injuries with a sturdy, canine-pleasant cleaner to cast off the odors that would enchantment to your home canine decrease lower back to the identical spot.

Timing

Watch out for the signs and symptoms and symptoms and signs and symptoms telling you that your puppy wishes to transport potty. Whining, sniffing, circling, barking, or scratching on the door are all apparent signs and signs and signs and symptoms and symptoms that your dog wishes to move. As a elegant rule, you need to flow for a toilet run first component inside the morning and remaining difficulty at night time time. Also, generally take your domestic canine out after it eats, liquids, finishes an indoor playing consultation, or wakes up from a snooze.

With very extra youthful dogs, you may need to take them out each 30-60 mins.

Crate training

Many canine owners shy away at the concept of confining their little puppies in a crate. However,

a crate will assist you to spot the signs and symptoms and signs and symptoms and signs and symptoms on the same time as your puppy wants to go, making it easy to teach your canine to maintain it till you open the crate and permit it out. Make first-rate that the crate is big sufficient to your dog to rise up, lie down, and flip round, but not so massive that they may be capable of use one of the corners as a lavatory.

Don't take too extended to allow your property canine out, otherwise, it'll lose manage and might even get the idea that it's adequate to soil its living area. If this takes area, it's going to probably expect that it's k to soil your residing space, too. If you're the use of the crate for added than hours instantly, attach a dispenser to the crane to make certain that it has get right of entry to to easy water.

Paper education

Paper schooling is possibly the maximum handy housebreaking method for busy canine owners but this selection comes with one complex issue. Ideally, your home canine might learn how to preserve it interior and best do its enterprise organisation outside. Paper and domestic dog pads enhance the two opposing components on the equal time, which can be confusing on your pup if you decide to take it out of doors later whilst it grows up. However, in case you're incapable of taking your canine out severa times an afternoon, paper training may be a appropriate possibility, as prolonged as it receives used to an authorized spot at home.

House soiling is one of the most crucial reasons why many puppies grow to be in shelters or at the streets. Very few pet proprietors are willing to location up with a canine that destroys their rugs and floors, or leaves a nasty mess for them to smooth after an extended, tiring day. This is why it's important to start potty training your home dog early right now to save you terrible behavior from forming and turning into harder to govern within the destiny. Don't worry if there are setbacks; housebreaking calls for consistency, staying power, and staying power. As prolonged as you maintain at it, your doggy will in the end study.

How to Crate Train Your Puppy

Crates are typically used for transporting dogs from one region to every distinctive, however they will do masses extra than that. By providing a non-public, enclosed space, a crate takes benefit of a dog's natural instincts to be a den animal, supplying it with a stable canine lair where it can be cushty.

Not first-rate will your doggy be stable in its crate but your sanity and peace of mind can also be preserved when you can relaxation confident that your domestic canine isn't chewing up your fixtures or soiling your private home at the identical time as you're out. However, your home canine isn't probable to get used to the idea of a crate proper away. To make crate training a piece less hard for you, we've assembled the excellent tips from the devoted canine professionals.

Choose the right crate

Before you get began on crate training, you need to first recognize the manner to choose out the fantastic one on your home canine. The very idea behind why crates are used for housebreaking is because dogs are very easy creatures by means of nature and they don't like a urine-soaked residing vicinity any more than you do. This is likewise why the size of the crate subjects the maximum. Find a nicely-ventilated crate that's just large enough to your domestic dog to stand up, lie down, and flip spherical simply.

If the crate is just too massive, your dog might imagine that it's good enough to apply one of the corners as a relaxation room and take a seat with no problem faraway from the mess, that can encourage future injuries all through the residence. And if it's too small, your dog will not enjoy staying in it and this can probably make potty schooling lots more difficult for you in go returned.

Remember that the crate has to residence your doggy as it grows, so pick one that's appropriate for the predicted whole-grown length of your canine and use a divider to address your pup's smaller duration inside the period in-between. Alternatively, you can purchase a crate that carries an adjustable partition that you could adapt to the size of your home canine as it grows.

Get your doggy to like the crate

For a successful education technique, the crate should typically be associated to 3 detail exquisite. Make the crate more inviting through lining it with blankets and putting a few toys inner. Place the crate in a immoderate-pastime vicinity which includes the living room, in that you and the opportunity family people spend quite a few time. When you first introduce your pup to the crate, inspire it to enter with the aid of way of going on to its diploma and speaking to it in a satisfied voice.

You also can trap it in by using way of losing a few teats close to the crate, then go away some just in the door, and subsequently, toss some all the manner inner. If it though refuses to head in at the start, that's o.K., don't force it to go into. Whether it takes a few minutes or a few days, preserve tempting it with treats till it willingly walks inner.

Gradually condition your doggy to get used to the crate

Introduction

At first, deliver your domestic dog to the crate for 10-minute breaks and provide it motivating treats or distracting toys whilst it's miles going interior. Once your domestic dog is inner, take a seat down down silently close to the crate for about five minutes after which depart the room for a couple of minutes. When you come back, sit down quietly for a fast on the equal time as and then allow your domestic dog out of the crate. Repeat this approach as a minimum two times a day and frequently growth the period of time you depart it within the crate.

Association

To get your domestic dog to companion lavatory time with crate time, take it for a walk every time it comes out of the crate. Once you attain the volume where your domestic canine stays lightly in its crate for half of-hour with you out of sight, you could begin leaving it indoors whilst you're long long past for brief time intervals. Keep letting your home canine inside the crate for quick intervals now and again whilst you're domestic so it doesn't partner crate time with abandonment.

Sleep

Once your home dog is used to being on my own in its crate for multiple hours with out getting demanding, you may allow it sleep there at night time. This can take days or possibly weeks depending in your dog's temperament among different factors however the most essential issue is to face up to the temptation to hurry the conditioning approach. Learning takes time however if you live affected person and steady, your own home canine will in the end discover ways to love its crate for destiny years.

When crating your home dog in a single day, it's usually recommended which you positioned the crate for your bed room or on hallway outdoor your bed room door as it will probable need to transport outside at some degree inside the night time time time and you need that allows you to pay attention it at the equal time as it whines to be set free. Always make certain that your domestic dog has get right of get entry to to to clean water while you're leaving it in its crate.

Never go away your puppy in its crate all day

A crate isn't a paranormal pass for potty education. If it's no longer used well, the crate will enjoy like a jail as opposed to a shelter in your canine and this will make it feel stressful, trapped, and abandoned. If your pup feels ignored, it'll most possibly act out in pass again.

Dogs need severa toilet breaks as well as play and feeding instances. Young puppies, in particular, shouldn't be saved crated for extra than 3 or 4 hours at a time due to the truth they might't manage their bladder and bowels prolonged intervals of time.

Crate training your home dog may also moreover take some time and attempt however while you get the hang of it, it's going to are to be had in reachable in quite some conditions. Whether you want to limit your doggy's get right of entry to to the residence till it learns all of the house policies otherwise you need to take it to the vet at the same time as shielding your vehicle's valuable seats, the previous guidelines can assist make your dog's crate revel in hundreds more first-rate. Remember that even in case your pup's crate is its den, sincerely as you wouldn't want to spend most of some time in a room, your dog shouldn't spend maximum of its time in a crate.

Chapter 4: How To Bond With Your Puppy

Bonding with your domestic dog is one of the maximum vital things that can rise up. Bonding is not notable a training itself, bonding is a few component a superb deal deeper. There is a real energetic connection in case you improve your pup with love. You can train a canine and educate all of them types of tricks however great thru love can the doggy continuously discover a way over again to you.

Love is a kingdom of thoughts. There might be times you can revel in you have "fallen out of affection" together with your doggy much like the primary time they nip you or once they stubbornly disobey you. Love is a willpower. Ask your pup what love is. They recognize. Dogs set the equal vintage for love. You leave them by myself all day at the same time as you visit paintings or pass play and they'll be heartbroken, maybe outraged. But the immediate they see you, all is forgiven. They welcome you lower back with loving paws and a large slobbery lick at the nose. No extra love exists than the love a dog has for their human.

I actually have seen scared dogs, competitive puppies, or very shy ones. It isn't necessarily their genetic fault, however as an alternative a replica of its proprietor. Some of those behaviors can be steady, a number of them faded however some will never vanish, relying on the dog's character and the impact of its owner. Therefore, there may be a mindset and attributes you need to boom so that you can decorate and train the suitable doggy accomplice.

Mindset and Character of a splendid puppy proprietor

Patient: Great pup owner must be affected man or woman. There can be instances your pup won't listen flawlessly. There might be times your pup disobeys you or maybe does a few harm. Patience is the key and understanding that this stuff seem and it is a part of the technique makes the scenario less difficult.

Committed: You need to be committed to being the great feasible determine for your doggy. In appropriate times, and in awful instances, you must be there for them.

Responsible: Having a home dog isn't always handiest a laugh. There are pretty some duties that take vicinity and also you need to take rate of them. Vaccination, simple fitness care, walking, feeding, and providing each day glowing water are requirements for a puppy's healthy increase.

Accessible: Honestly, adopting a home dog virtually to be domestic by myself all the time is not the awesome concept. You or a number of your own family members ought to constantly be to be had, in close to environment to the doggy. A home canine wants to sense the presence of different people and they'll bond the maximum with the person who will love and spend greater time with them.

Trustworthy: Generally, don't forget isn't given; it's earned. That isn't always normally the case with dogs regardless of the truth that. Unless you provide them a motive now not to take into account you, it commonly comes instilled in them. They will bear in mind you to attend to them, love, feed, water, and educate them. Don't allow them to down, being trusted is a privilege past degree.

Leader of the Pack: You've likely heard of % order. Dogs, like wolves and plenty of different animals, are social animals installation with a "pecking order." They have a "% mentality" that incorporates submission and dominance. By setting up your self, the owner and teacher, due to the fact the % leader, your dog will glaringly publish; it's miles in their genes to accomplish that. Whether you are a "%" advocate or now not, there is reality to the notion, as even our children are taught to conform with order with the useful resource of way of authority. Call it what you may, but you may need to set up your management with love or your pup may additionally very well expect they will be the pinnacle of the circle of relatives.

How to bond together in conjunction with your house canine

Spending time collectively is the entirety nearly approximately any courting and the greater, the higher. The dating among you and your new doggy isn't always any exception. The warmness, fuzzy feeling you get at the equal time as you pup them and the moments you percentage looking into each different's eyes units the scene, but it doesn't decide it.

When you first convey your domestic dog into your own home, you could want to spend nice time together. If you could, take a few days off artwork or school in order that the two of you could bond. If that isn't viable, bringing them domestic for your day or days off is better than in the course of the busiest time of your week but as I stated earlier, it's miles generally better if any character is inside the home dog's presence maximum of the time, as a minimum, the primary month.

Keep in thoughts that, as mentioned earlier, your doggy has never been a domestic dog before. They don't have any idea the manner to behave, what to do, or what to expect. It is as a lot as you to permit them to recognize. Assure them and reassure them. When they cry at night, they may be most probable lacking Their mother and siblings.

Giving them love and safety doesn't imply you need to bend the recommendations. If you have got established the truth that Sweetie Pie gained't be sharing your bed, gently tuck them back in after they be troubled, truely as you'll a little one. If the state of affairs receives out of hand, you may must exercising a hint "difficult love." Let them yelp, but acquire this with durations of loving pats and sort phrases.

Talking to your home dog, taking them for walks, and certainly spending time together are treasured for putting a agency foundation, similar to with human parenting. Yes, you examine it proper, the more you verbally speak to your domestic dog, the extra they will seize without delay to topics, and the closer the two of you becomes. Just as you do with a toddler, say the names of factors like, "ball", "water" and "stroll." You can be surprised how fast they research the names of people, locations, and matters. Sing to them too; puppies love a first rate music, despite the fact that they may howl in case you sing off-key.

Puppies are truely playful, curious, and active. Those inclinations are going to be a laugh most of the time, but a good manner to keep your friend regular and protected, you want to help them set up obstacles. The awesome tip to start with is that you need to recall your doggy like you'll a human toddler. Treat them as though they had been an infant or a infant. Here are a few pup schooling suggestions that you could use to teach your domestic canine the whole lot they want to recognise to begin the journey of turning into your high-quality pal.

Puppy Proofing Your Home

One of the primary subjects you will need to do with a modern day home dog is to pup-evidence your house. Set up gates and close to doorways, preserving the domestic dog restricted to a specific place. Your little dog might be no longer housebroken but, and you do now not need to clean up messes all at some stage in your property. Keeping the home canine inner your form of sight for the number one few weeks is important. You'll also want to choose up some thing it sincerely is at the floor. Puppies are famous for chewing up garments, shoes, your little one's favourite toy, and some thing else they are capable of get their keen little mouths round.

Treats and Rewards

Everyone, together with puppies, loves treats. You can use those as a reward for appropriate behavior. Dog treats are to be had all flavors, sizes, and specialties. Soft, meaty treats are very appealing to most dogs, and having a prepared deliver on hand will assist your home dog short have a have a look at what behaviors are favored and rewarded. Puppies typically love treats with cheese, peanut butter, or meat flavor. Select small treats in area of huge ones that require a whole lot of chewing. The trick with schooling is to use quick, first-rate reinforcement and small, chunk-sized treats as a really perfect reward to your home canine but you may all discover about it later on this ebook.

Drop a deal with into the secure haven if you have one so one can entice your canine internal. Provide a cope with anytime the puppy goes to the relaxation room outside or sits and rolls over whilst commanded. Don't deliver your canine treats for no cause, or this will confuse the state of affairs and they won't understand they will be being rewarded. Make certain it's miles a appropriate dog deal with that you're offering as nicely.

Your rewards need to also range. If you constantly offer them a cope with following a voice command, they will associate the command with meals. If they don't need or want food, then he'll refuse the command. Instead, if your reward includes giving them a address, soothing them, playing with them, or petting them, then they apprehend that they will get a few type of praise while following the command. This manner a pup will discover ways to always pay hobby to your instructions now not handiest looking beforehand to a few kind of address. Anything that produces wonderful feelings which incorporates gambling or petting them counts.

Communicating Your Intentions Clearly

There's no longer something incorrect with explicitly telling your domestic dog "no", quality that it frequently fails to provide sufficient facts. Instead, you can inform them what you need. Dogs do no longer typically generalize well, so if the dog jumps on a person in pleasure and you say "no", they'll jump better or exchange path. A better opportunity may be to teach them to sit down down. Telling them what you want allows avoid confusion.

One of the maximum crucial errors at the equal time as trying to find to apply voice commands is using too many phrases. Your canine can associate terms, but it takes a while. You'll need a word that is to the detail. Finish getting to know one command earlier than shifting immediately to each different. If you circulate immediately to unique commands too short, then your canine can also moreover get careworn.

Be Consistent

You should be regular in case you want your pup to be regular. You can't paintings for an hour on a sit down command after which simply now not take in their education over again for every week or . You need to paintings at the same command every day till they get it proper.

Establish bodily sports together with your domestic dog, which includes ordinary feeding instances, stroll, and play instances, and rest room breaks. Stick along side your workout routines and this will assist boost up the method. It's not just about schooling commands both. A routine in your domestic dog will assist them get up while you do, play on the identical time as you experience as a first rate deal as it, and devour even as you are capable of feed them. This manner you aren't rearranging your time desk to take care of your home dog. Instead, you'll be education them to artwork on your time table in order that they artwork with you.

If you do no longer need your own home canine to leap on human beings while they come through the the the front door, you need to boost that expectation on every occasion. Allowing the puppy to jump throughout your sister, however no longer your neighbor will motive confusion. Use the "take a seat down" or "stay" or "heel" command (you will examine later on this e book) to get your puppy's hobby and do it whenever. Be constant due to the fact inconsistencies will only confuse them and boom the schooling gadget.

Use Repetition

Repetition is high in canine schooling. Dogs have a look at from repetition. The high-quality command will become related with pleasant conduct within the home canine's mind. It wishes to be accomplished with precision and right timing. If the doggy performs your command, reward it proper now. If not, overlook approximately about it and strive once more till it's far completed successfully.

Be Patient

Even extra staying strength, however YES, it is a important exquisite. Don't allow your self to get aggravated or impatient sooner or later of the schooling system – both with your self or together collectively along with your new doggy. It will make an effort to accomplish all of the goals you have got got set in your new pal and if you want to get the grasp of your domestic dog's unique man or woman, likes, and the techniques and rewards that paintings nice for your puppy.

Give your pup time to recognize new instructions. They maximum likely won't study it the number one couple of times when you teach them. Repeat antique commands in new training sessions, in order that they don't forget about them. The interest span of a dog is pretty short, so hold your classes common but short in period, otherwise, your domestic canine turns into bored.

Never get impatient along side your domestic dog and in no way name them to you in case you are going to punish them – all on the way to do is train them that coming to you isn't an brilliant thing. The handiest manner you do it at the same time as you spot undesirable conduct is to go back to the house dog, call them their call to get their hobby, and supply a modern day command, if finished effectively, praise straight away saying "Good boy/girl". Keep your voice enterprise business enterprise but mild, and in no way allow any frustration creep into it.

Train Yourself

When you introduce a present day dog into your own family and your lifestyles, you're no longer virtually education the house dog. You're schooling your self as properly. Your life goes to need to exchange, and also you want to be organized for it and willing to evolve. Sleeping in till midday on the weekends isn't always an desire when you have a home dog that desires to be walked and fed. Taking off for a spontaneous excursion appears like fun, however first, you may need to make preparations for the domestic dog. Working with the canine to be calm and quiet while buddies and family go to takes hundreds of electricity and a willingness to recognize in there for the long term.

Possible motives of not bonding together at the side of your pup

Possible causes of now not bonding in conjunction with your puppy are the opposite of what you have to do to nicely bond in conjunction with your home canine. Not being available, being impatient, and punishing the pup inside the wrong manner and wrong time.

One of my clients, Trisha, had multiple problems together collectively along with her new home canine. She found a male Staffordshire terrier and called him Tyson. On our first appointment, she cautioned me she accompanied this breed in clean terms because she clearly loved it. She did not do any research beforehand, she had been given advice from her buddies who had a dog on a manner to train him.

Because Trisha become a younger, busy woman living on her very non-public, spending some of time at paintings, she

wasn't to be had for the domestic dog as she need to be. Anytime she have been given yet again domestic, there were excrements everywhere within the area due to the fact she didn't need to lock the puppy in a crate. The trouble become that she punished that doggy for the excrement thru manner of pulling their fur a piece.

Sometimes even as she were given again home, her garments were chewed-up in pieces because of the truth the doggy have been given bored. Of path, the domestic dog end up punished for that too. When Trisha became jogging in the direction of obedience schooling with Tyson, after a couple of instances of commanding the phrase "Sit" and failing to perform that, she bent over and hugged him pronouncing "You are my little satan, aren't you?" and kissed him.

I knew right away what grow to be wrong. We started out out out fixing all the ones topics proper away. First, because of the fact there couldn't be some exceptional character concerned, we brilliant had one opportunity. Train her pup to live most effective in a unmarried room.

Trisha decided to smooth up considered one in every of her rooms and set up a pet gate, leaving not something else besides food, water, and masses of chewing toys for her little satan. Because a puppy needs to be walked greater regularly than an character canine, her brother should prevent by way of the use of way of and take Tyson for a walk. That didn't save you Tyson from having a piece twist of fate every so often but greater human touch among Tyson and Trisha's brother changed into created and this is continuously useful.

Since then, Tyson wasn't punished anymore due to the fact that in reality failed to make sense. Firstly, the domestic dog can't hyperlink the punishment with the twist of destiny that took place an hour in the past. Now you're punishing a home dog and that they do not recognize the cause at the back of the punishment. Secondly, as and you may look at in this book, we're elevating a pup with love. We don't punish our puppies. We notify them and then accurate them thru commanding desired conduct, however clearly now not bodily punishing them.

Lastly, if your dog does no longer time and again pay interest on your commands, you do not pup him announcing "You are my little satan, aren't you? Why? Because that complements the house dog's disobedience. If the home canine again and again doesn't pay attention, you both forget about about it or permit it glide certainly. Maybe the domestic dog might be worn-out inside the meantime, distracted thru a few factor else, otherwise you don't speak virtually to them. Either manner, there's a impartial reaction and you pass on and attempt later.

Since then, Trisha and Tyson have advanced a much higher, greater healthful, and extra data relationship. If you have got got the right records, matters drift thousands a great deal less tough. There are masses of conditions and relationships that don't pass well. If that takes location, we should never blame the home dog, however take a look at ourselves first. We are accountable for the improvement of our domestic dog; the man or woman and conduct the domestic dog will very very own within the future is actually from our contribution.

So now you have got a superb perception of the manner to connect to your new pup. You have observed out what mindset it takes to be a brilliant domestic canine determine and you realize the manner the home canine feels approximately being in a contemporary home with new human beings. You also realise what are the reasons of now not bonding along with your home dog and a way to prevent that before it takes place. In the following bankruptcy, we will talk the way to pick out the proper breed for you, and I will damage down unique canine breeds so that you will be extra confident in choosing the right wholesome for you. Let's get to it.

Chapter 5: Choosing The Right Breed Of Puppy

You've made the selection to transport beforehand and bring a present day day doggy into your lifestyles and home. It's interesting and happy, and it is able to be tough to be affected character whilst you're so prepared to deliver that new little package deal of pride domestic.

BUT, dashing out to the nearby domestic dog keep, or locating out the classifieds and rushing off to buy the primary little home canine that chews for your shoelaces may be a horrible idea for such a lot of reasons!

There are over 340 diagnosed dog breeds that fall into one in all six training - toy, carrying, hound, terrier, operating, and herding.

However, it's very vital to hold in thoughts that each breed has its very personal very precise 'appearance', personality and wishes, and so do you and your own family contributors. Let's have a check the pinnacle

12 Family dog breeds so you can get a revel in of similarities or differences specifically dogs.

Top 12 Family Dog Breeds

1. Labrador Retriever

Labrador Retriever is one in each of my favorites! Highly clever, awesome-natured, very willing, and keen to delight. These active puppies have an first rate, dependable temperament and are superb, wonderful with children, and equable with one of a kind dogs. They can perform all forms of hints.

2. Golden Retriever

These are lovely, well-mannered, intelligent puppies with excellent appeal. They are with out trouble educated, generally affected character, and mild with children. Fantastic member of the family.

three. Beagle

The Beagle is loving, candy, and mild, satisfied to peer every person, greeting them with a wagging tail. It is sociable, brave, and realistic.

four. German Shepherd

German Shepherd dogs are quite devoted, and brave. They will no longer expect twice approximately giving their lives for his or her human percent. They have a immoderate studying potential. German Shepherds like to be near their households, however can be cautious of strangers. This breed dreams its human beings and ought to not be left remoted for lengthy intervals of time.

five. Boxer

The Boxer is satisfied, excessive-lively, playful, curious, and energetic. Highly sensible, eager, and short to have a take a look at, the Boxer is a notable canine for competitive obedience. It is constantly at the bypass and bonds very closely with the family. Loyal and affectionate, Boxers are recounted for the way they get alongside so properly with youngsters.

6. Bulldog

The Bulldog is some of the gentlest of dogs. Just the identical it will see off any intruder. It is described as a totally affectionate and reliable animal, moderate with youngsters, but recognised for its braveness and its wonderful guarding capabilities. Bulldogs are very a super deal a human beings's dog, looking for human interest and loving each bit they are capable of get!! A lot of human hobby is wanted for the breed's happiness.

7. Dachshund

You might realize this canine as a "sausage dog". Long body, quick legs, . Some would possibly probably have a funny appearance but, Dachshunds are wonderful tourists. This little canine dreams an proprietor who's acquainted with a manner to be their percent leader or they'll take over the house, and begin to attempt to inform the owner what to do.

eight. Pitbull

Pitbulls are very dependable, lovely dogs. They also are pretty defensive in their home and what they view as their territory. This can make them a piece possessive and aggressive. A Pitbull needs stability, firmness, and regular education a awesome manner to be well-behaved within the domestic. These dogs are very athletic and want quite some movement and sports activities.

9. Staffordshire terrier

The Staffordshire Terrier is an sensible, brave, and determined dog, which makes them splendid watchdogs. This breed isn't always for every body, but. Very similar to Pitbull, Staffordshire Terrier is an athletic breed that desires to be loaded with sports activities.

10. Goldendoodle

A Goldendoodle is a pleasant, lively dog that loves to play and be engaged. They love hobby and will thrive in an active circle of relatives. A Goldendoodle makes a excellent own family pup. Very lovable and passionate breed.

eleven. Jack Russell Terrier

Jack Russell Terrier loves to play and loves humans. This breed is right with youngsters and special dogs, however won't do well with cats. They are clever, a laugh-loving, and affectionate.

12. Border Collie

Border Collie is an clever, lively, and eager-to-please dog. This breed within reason trainable and makes a exquisite associate for any form of family. Border Collies are lively, outgoing, and very satisfactory puppies. They will do properly with kids within the proper situation. They want everyday exercising or they may begin to get themselves into hassle! They also can carry out an exceptional quantity of recommendations, and they will be getting to know very quickly.

Dogs variety in masses of factors, no longer truely in character. Size, top, and weight play a number one function in maturity. Therefore it is very essential to be clear of what you want to deal with; because as a home dog, any breed is viable due to its size, however as the domestic dog grows, there is probably conditions that you'll be wanting to deal with.

Before you pick out out your new home dog, it's far crucial to mirror your very personal existence too. Sometimes we would like a specific breed but that may not go with the flow nicely with our way of life or manner of dwelling, probable causing extra problems than pleasures. It is right to recognize what to search for while choosing a domestic dog and here are 10 crucial problems from the owner's angle whilst choosing a domestic dog.

eight Important Considerations When Choosing A New Puppy

Do you have got children?

If so, then you definitely surely'll need to choose out a breed that has the right temperament for kids. Your kids can even must be dog-fine — prepare for the more steps it takes to train them to train the canine, and to respect their location.

The majority of puppies will get collectively with children truly top notch if they may be raised with them. However, a few breeds have a defensive streak in them and can emerge as aggressive with youngsters who get too close to at mealtime, or competitive with youngsters they've got in no way met.

These breeds will possibly see the youngsters as being under themselves in the "p.C. Order" and can try to dominate them.

Some puppies will patiently put up with little kids who pull their ears or by manner of risk poke them within the eyes, at the same time as others will now not and can nip or bite once more in protection.

So if you need a dog who is tremendous with kids keep away from breeds that could have a dominance streak or which have short tempers.

Do You Already Have Other Dogs In Your Home?

Remember, all puppies, even domesticated ones, have a p.C. Mentality. Bringing a brand new doggy into "your %" includes more steps. Watch your capability puppy on the secure haven to look how they get along side the opposite puppies. If the domestic canine is combative there, it's a completely sturdy indicator that it might be combative at your own home as properly.

Puppies with Coats and Shedding

Dogs with long coats require every day brushing otherwise their coats will become raveled and tangled. Not only can it damage your dog in the event that they have tangled and disheveled hair, however it will moreover grow to be grimy and they will look shaggy and unsightly in case you do not regularly brush their coat.

So preserve in thoughts that during case you pick out out a breed with an extended coat you will each need to get it clipped frequently if you want to avoid brushing it so much, or if you pick to hold it lengthy or possibly medium period you could need to brush it every day.

Does Your Work Require A Lot Of Travel?

Do you need to excursion for art work or have an extended move back and forth? If so, do you've got were given help or are you capable of put money into assist at the equal time as you're away?

What Type of Lifestyle Do You Have – Active or Sedentary?

You need to be honest with yourself, due to the fact each type of canine has its very own needs and degree of care. Are you positive you're inclined to take your dog walking for 30-mins on a cold February morning? If you aren't too much for an prolonged, active stroll then bear in mind a breed that isn't too worrying. Adopting a Pitbull or Jack Russell Terrier may not be the awesome in shape for you.

Do You Live in a Home With a Yard or a Small Condo or Apartment?

That adorable little pup you have got your eye on may be small now, however will it increase right right right into a large, active canine? If so, likely you need to rethink your dream breed. Remember, despite the fact that, that even some smaller, more active puppies can soak up a whole lot of area (and strength) of their personal manner.

Can You Afford the home canine?

Bringing a current doggy into your existence and domestic calls for a determination similar to the dedication to be chargeable for a little one. This is a commitment that shouldn't be taken lightly.

It can variety with the aid of breed, but your domestic canine may want to turn out to be costing you from $600 to extra or much less $900 each 12 months — past what you paid for add-ons and to undertake them. So, in advance than you devote, make a fee variety and figure out what you could address. Also undergo in thoughts, a domestic dog received't be a pup all of the time. As they increase, they'll eat more and with a bit of luck will constantly be healthy so that you will in no way want to fear approximately high-priced veterinary payments.

Recurring veterinary bills?

There are initial fees which could consist of the subsequent - $2 hundred to spay or neuter — plus $a hundred and fifty for the number one exam, a few other $a hundred and fifty for vaccinations, $one hundred thirty for heartworm sorting out. It's clever to plot the manner you'll pay for ongoing hospital treatment. Put aside a similarly $210 for toy breeds and as an awful lot as $260 for a huge dog, and truly remember doggy scientific clinical medical health insurance. (The rate can variety nation to u.S.A., additionally this is the fee of time writing this ebook) Where To Find Your New Puppy

Essentially, you have got three options – You can visit a safe haven, touch a rescue institution, or visit a breeder.

Fortunately, the internet is an vital part of regular lifestyles and society. There are surely on-line web web sites that assist you to discover dogs which can be up for adoption.

Almost every county and the bigger town has a refuge run with the useful resource of the nearby government, further to others run with the aid of manner of nonprofit groups. Some may also have present day centers, and others can be extra fundamental however, in standard, puppies from shelters can have had photographs and possibly a few crucial education because those motive them to greater adoptable.

Don't be misled into thinking that shelters handiest have mutts and blended breeds. It is envisioned that 25 percent of puppies up for adoption are purebreds who have been given up for loads reasons.

Adopting From a Shelter

Before you go to a safe haven, you need to put together yourself emotionally as it's clean to get caught up and swept away via the usage of all of the ones adorable, pleading faces.

Here's What You Need To Know Before You Go

If possible, attempt to choose a safe haven this is near your house so you can without issue make numerous visits if you're having hassle selecting a domestic dog.

Ideally, you need to get a real feel of a home canine's individual. It's an superb concept to ignore a pup inside the starting, but stand or sit down close by, so you can get used in your presence and your fragrance.

If you face the canine or strive to talk to them, they ought to regulate to you, and you acquired't be capable of get to truly understand them.

Body language and power are very critical and you'll want to pay near attention to them. Ears perked up and tail held immoderate? That can also additionally signal an excited, dominant country, that you shouldn't praise with interest. Give interest to a submissive canine whose head is slightly down and whose tail is wagging however held halfway up.

Dogs that rush to the the front of the cage are displaying symptoms of anxiety, frustration, or dominance. A domestic dog that cowers behind the cage may additionally have shyness problems which could translate into worry-associated aggressiveness.

Try to slender your choice down to 2 or 3. Take each one for a quick leash walk and ask the safe haven employees about the home canine's personalities and conduct. Do they've got any health troubles, as an instance? Or have they been adopted and lower back? If so, why? Prepare your list of questions and get all of the way all the way down to a company.

Choosing a Good Breeder

As with in search of to choose out any company organisation, getting referrals is a fantastic useful aid. If people communicate nicely of a breeder, then that's a incredible signal that they deal with their animals and feature immoderate requirements. Some outstanding places to get referrals are vets, the American Kennel Club (AKC), and close by breed golf equipment.

A unique breeder may be capable of solution questions about the dog's ancestry (do not forget to invite approximately parents' and grandparents' temperaments. This will permit you to understand a great deal).

The energy diploma is important, so ensure to invite about it. Pay hobby to behavior. If a pup bounces off the partitions on the breeder's, he'll possibly do it at your property.

It's a awesome concept to invite the breeder for the touch records of various human beings who have accompanied puppies from them. Make sure you be conscious severa dogs, so you can locate the one you're maximum cushty — and nicely matched — with.

This is honestly critical — No particular breeder will ever will assist you to undertake a home dog that's greater youthful than eight weeks antique. A respectable breeder normally has the first rate interest of the puppy and the ultra-modern capacity proprietor. When deciding on a doggy from a refuge, breeder, or rescue organization, usually depend upon tremendous critiques and references.

Your puppy may be usual in any set of behavior you will please but that received't comply with one hundred% of the time. There are natural instincts and inherited dispositions that make your domestic canine particular. If you want to recognize who your doggy is inside the depth, optionally you can perform a set of those assessments.

Puppy Personality Testing

There isn't any "one length fits all" and character and temperament aren't solid in stone at starting.

However, the concept of "home canine trying out" with the aid of giving a puppy a few smooth checks has obtained recognition within the path of the dog global. One of the first-rate-recounted collection of exams is the "Volhard Test", that's called after the couple who standardized their personal finding out strategies to assist grow to be aware of a canine's character.

The practical cause inside the again of this type of test is to gauge a domestic dog's "dominance diploma", or how headstrong they're through nature. An noticeably ambitious canine is going to be a handful to teach, while on the alternative give up of the spectrum the very shy domestic canine—who may be startled with the useful aid of its private shadow— may be difficult to teach for specific motives.

Puppy character trying out moreover offers a feel of a pup's stage of hobby in people, which has an immediate impact on their trainability and the manner without hassle he'll emerge as a member of "your p.C.".

Age for Testing

Seven weeks—40-9 days to be real—is considered to be the appropriate age for a puppy to be evaluated far from the muddle. Except for a small quantity of located out conduct, a seven-week-vintage domestic dog is concept to be a clean slate, which means that testing right now is meant to offer a actual studying of their nature.

Puppy-Testing Situations

Of course, there are versions on how puppies can also reply to any of those "pop tests," however I include handiest ends of the spectrum: something in amongst is your judgment name. But within the case of very dominant or very submissive puppies, you may predict that they'll behave almost the identical manner in every state of affairs.

It's as a good deal as you whether or no longer you attempt some or all of those experiments, however try no longer to get too critical approximately them. Just use them as a baseline take a look at to get a trendy idea of the domestic dog's temperament.

The winning expertise is that you need to avoid any personality extremes in a domestic dog: now not the laid-decrease back pup, however now not the maximum ahead and pushy one, both. Other than that, attempt some of the little checks that follow—"Pop Tests for Pups," you may possibly name them—and notice which appeals to you as a way to get to recognize a pup rapid.

Puppy Testing Guidelines

•Use a room that is unusual to the dogs.

•Perform the tests while the dogs are at their most energetic.

•Puppies get a self guarantee increase from their clutter pals, so perform the test in my view.

Personality Test #1 - Shows whether or not or no longer or now not a canine accepts social domination

Bend down and firmly stroke from the home canine's head all of the manner all the way down to the pinnacle of their shoulders. A canine's head, neck, and shoulders are dominant regions: even as puppies meet, the better-ranking one will regularly placed their paw or chin during the withers (the ridge a number of the shoulder bones) of the alternative.

Ideally, a domestic dog will in all likelihood no longer object to this. They might possibly whine, wiggle, or stiffen for a second, but then he'll lighten up or even lick you.

A dominant home canine will probably item to your dominating stroking of them—they will growl or try to jump on you. They may also panic, war or freeze and not snap out of it.

Personality Test #2 - This check measures hobby and eagerness approximately human beings. Do they enjoy human affection enough to paintings for it in training?

Bend down, clap your hands, but don't name the puppy right away—just watch. Ideally, a puppy comes right over, and will live with you, wagging its tail. A dominant domestic dog may additionally chew at you or wander off disinterested.

Personality Test #3 - Call the Puppy to You: crouch down, clap your hands, whistle, sound encouraging

Bend down, and open your fingers for the maximum welcoming role. A dominant domestic canine would probably forget about you, or come at once at you and nip, bounce or come across you after they get there.

Personality Test #4 - Will They Follow You?

Stroke the domestic dog, walk away, then see how conveniently they agree to. Ideally, a home canine follows you.

A dominant domestic canine follows, however so near that they get underfoot and can even try and chunk at your ft or garments.

Personality Test #5- Hold

 the Puppy Off the Floor: Cradle Your Hands Under Their Stomach

What does the pup do after they haven't any manipulate and you've got desired manage?

Gently carry them some inches off the ground and keep the place for fifteen seconds.

Ideally, a domestic dog struggles a bit, then relaxes in your hands.

A dominant doggy will conflict and fight and can bark, whine or attempt to chew your fingers.

Personality Test #6: Sit down and preserve the domestic dog on their once more for your lap: stroke their stomach, speak reassuringly

What is their reaction to being lightly limited?

Ideally, a doggy will war in short and then lighten up.

A dominant pup will thrash around to get off its once more and can vocalize or bite.

Personality Test #7: -Retrieving. Set the doggy on the ground, get their interest with the aid of way of waving a ball or toy, after which roll it within the course of the floor. Make enthusiastic, encouraging, "Come on woman/boy!" noises to carry it once more.

Ideally, a domestic canine will chase the object, play with it and likely even deliver it decrease lower again to you in case you clap your arms and whistle. They will will let you take it away with out an excessive amount of objection.

A dominant home dog will chase the object and take off with it, ignoring you at the same time as you try to recall them. If you try and take it lower back they received't relinquish it and may growl.

So there you skip. You have already observed some aspect, have not you? In this chapter you have got found out about unique tempers examined with the aid of dogs, you placed out what to don't forget even as choosing a home dog to be the proper match and you have got were given discovered how to test a domestic dog for its diploma of dominance which may be beneficial on your training endeavors. You moreover recognize wherein to go to pick out your property canine, and what to search for. You are all set to make topics occur, now topics begin to get thrilling due to the reality in the subsequent chapter you are about to discover the tremendous way to transition your private home dog from muddle for your new domestic, how your first day collectively ought to seem like, and hundreds more. Are you organized? So turn the net web page.

Chapter 6: Easy Transitioning Of A Puppy From Litter To New Home

Puppies are tiny, defenseless, and an extended way away from their mother, so they want greater care and a watchful eye to make sure that they increase healthfully. You might be a chunk crushed and forced as to how exactly you must pass about doing so, and it's handiest herbal that you're feeling this way. With a few studies and cautious planning, even though, you'll surely end up a skillful fur-determine very quickly.

Bringing a brand new puppy domestic is a cute deal with for the whole circle of relatives, one which could considerably brighten each person's day. Since granting a secure and loving home for a doggy is not any small feat, there are some matters to recollect earlier of time. You want to supply your puppy into a puppy-equipped surroundings. Here is a listing of things you may keep in thoughts looking for.

Prepare Essentials For Your Puppy

Dog-evidence fence

Canines are obviously curious creatures. The accurate news is, in the occasion that they ever discover their way out, they'll probable be able to take a look at the perfume back domestic. However, there's masses to worry approximately beyond the fence of your private home that could seriously injure your dog, and in some immoderate instances, result in its dying.

If you don't have a fence right now, don't supply your dog domestic inside the desire of maintaining it as a strictly indoor domestic canine. Even if you stroll your canine each morning, you're though going to need it to wander approximately on your yard for a few slight solar publicity, and to offer it extra area to discover and get enough exercise whilst not having to be on a leash.

Dogs also have a propensity to become bored with out issues, so get right of entry to to the outside will allow them to observe your associates and possibly even chase some squirrels. Don't fear, it's now not going that they'll seize any of them.

Another reason you need to get a fence is that it permits your first-rate buddy to freely get frequent bathroom breaks. This is specially crucial even as it's even though a home canine; you'll need to educate it in which it's adequate to move potty, otherwise you'll have lots to clean up on a every day basis.

Just keep in thoughts that obtaining a fence does not replace taking your canine on a walk. Dogs want to be walked every day for a alternate of environment, an unique sufficient quantity of exercise, and some intellectual stimulation. This additionally allows you bond collectively with your new puppy and offers it a few component to appearance in advance to every day.

Pet gates

When you're adopting a more youthful pup, you're going to want to hold the nosy little furball a ways from components of your home that might be volatile for it to discover, or some other place which you'd want to keep smooth and tidy. Canines are curious and messy, and any room they get right of access to may also emerge as being state of affairs to 3 chewed-up devices or broken vases.

There are gates specially designed for pets, however a few are so low that your property dog can discover ways to soar over them. Make positive the gates you cross for are every immoderate and sturdy enough.

I endorse you get the ones installation at a couple of entrances; despite the fact that, you shouldn't preserve them closed usually. They may be a first-rate way to location your canine not to interrupt you at the equal time as you're cooking or consuming. For the number one few months, assume your canine to bark and wail on the closed gate. It can be heartbreaking, however finally, your dog will study even as and in which it is able to get admission to regions in your home.

The opportunities are endless in terms of wherein you can install home dog gates, however I would possibly endorse in the direction of overusing them. Dogs anticipate to be handled as part of the circle of relatives. If you limit their get right of get entry to to to to multiple areas for prolonged durations of time, this moreover limits the time you spend along side your dog, that could take a toll on their intellectual fitness. Use the gates carefully, at the same time as you actually have to.

Chew toys

Think of chewing toys as pacifiers for toddlers. In their teething segment, dogs will both bite at the severa toys which you provide them, or they'll chew holes through your furnishings. There's number one/3 choice.

Chewing for developing puppies is similar to an itch that wants to be scratched, and it lets in them increase healthful enamel fast. However, that's now not to say that truely-grown puppies will save you using their chew toys. Wild dog naturally exert an entire lot of strive on the identical time as chewing through the flesh and bones of their prey—a herbal intuition that canned or dry food does now not satiate. Because your canine doesn't go out to are looking for for, it needs to discover a few factor else to bite on apart from prey.

Your options are infinite, and your choices actually rely on your dog. Most puppies, particularly puppies, revel in squeaky toys because they mimic squealing prey. It may additionally sound ugly, but it's pleasant intuition. You'll most probable need to offer your domestic dog with some of toys to pick out out out from.

Bigger plush toys might be their favourite to from time to time bite on, and moreover use as snuggle pillows once they nap. Bone-shaped squeaky toys are usually terrific distractions to bypass the time, or to enjoy a few exceptional playtime with you.

If you'll depart your dog unaccompanied for a few hours, the great toy to maintain it entertained with is a rubber bite treat toy, which can be complete of treats that ooze out of the toy when bit or squeezed. This additionally mimics a searching revel in, to be able to preserve your dog's instincts satiated, and will, in turn, help hold your doggy nicely-behaved.

There are also flavored toys, which double as toothbrushes in your domestic dog. These toys are specifically designed with clean bristles that clean your canine's teeth as it chews on the toy. They're excellent for a few extra dental care, however don't forget that they're able to't update an extensive teeth brushing ordinary. Some dogs are also finicky when it comes to reasonably-priced rubber that smells artificial. Opt for a flavored toy to make it extra appealing for your dog.

Food and water accessories

You have to spend money on a few strong and easy-to-clean food and water bowls as short as you could. Growing puppies have extensive appetites and also you need to make sure that you have the proper gear to be had to feed them regularly. It's truely beneficial to get a reasonably huge water bowl, too, as all dogs want smooth access to easy, easy water always.

Furthermore, you need to placed your puppy on a food plan advocated thru the vet as they will want to alter their meal plans constant with any particular issues or ailments presently traumatic your doggy.

An automated meals dispenser could be your pleasant pal (aside from your bushy companion) if you spend long hours at art work every day. Even in case you feed your dog as soon as you get again domestic, it's best to time desk timed feedings to your pet, specially for the cause that dogs virtually thrive on ordinary.

Many dog feeders can be timed to regulate your domestic dog's consuming schedule, and also you get to pick out out how lots you want to feed on a each day basis, as nicely. This may also even help in case your dog has an inclination to wake you up early in the morning, disturbing to be fed.

Feeders can paintings with moist or dry meals relying on the version, and exceptional producers cater to great sizes.

Timed 12-meal computerized feeders are taken into consideration the super and healthiest possibility for small or medium-sized dogs. This manner, in vicinity of eating massive meals, they're fed 12 smaller food at some degree in the day. The sluggish feed mode slowly dispenses meals over the course of 15 mins to save you your canine from vomiting, which generally takes vicinity at the same time as puppies eat too speedy.

But that doesn't imply that the device gets to pick while and the way your dog eats. If you need to set an ingesting time table to your dog for your personal phrases for clinical motives, there's a direct feed mode that lets in you to choose out out the part of food served as well.

Whatever dispenser you pick out for your dog, make sure you are taking out the tray or bowl to smooth it every day.

Dog residence

Dog house becomes extra applicable even as your property dog turns preferably 6 months antique. If you have got a residence with a outside and plan to keep your canine freely out of doors, take into account constructing a canine house. Dogs should typically be allowed to head returned indoors every time they need to, but if they often spend time in your outside (and that they probable will), it's exceptional to bring together a comfortable canine house for them.

For starters, this creates a region for them that they experience is their private. Just like your circle of relatives participants have a room in their personal, a dog residence may be your puppy's non-public region. Dog homes can also guard your pets from heat strokes; but, if it's even pretty hot for you outside, it's probable too warmness to your dog. Make exceptional that a few thing canine door you have got were given established may be locked while critical, so you can maintain your pal interior even as the weather conditions aren't pleasant.

You don't need to spend loads of bucks on custom-made canine homes that healthy the outdoor layout of your private home. Any frequently taking place den crafted from white cedar may be quite long lasting, and additionally steady to your canine. White cedar is also known as stained white timber, and the cause why it makes the right material for dog homes is that it's actually non-poisonous for pets and offers off a nice fragrance even though wet.

Aside from being an aesthetically attractive addition for your outdoor, it's moreover proof against excessive climate changes in addition to pests that would infest your lawn, so that you can rest assured that your dog can be stable underneath its little sloped roof.

If you're going to make your buy online, ensure you pick out the proper size. Dogs, in tremendous, revel in cushty regions, so some component too commodious in your fur infant isn't endorsed. Whatever you pick out, I propose you get one with ground panels, so your canine doesn't have to take a sleep on a wet lawn.

Grooming package deal

You want to at the least have a primary grooming kit at domestic, even in case you plan to often take your dog to a professional groomer.

Grooming isn't just about retaining your canine looking lovely. Trimming a dog's fur and nails often is sanitary and helps you notice any symptoms and signs of potential infections or ailments. Grooming your puppy often may even decrease coat and pores and pores and skin troubles like ordinary scratching, rashes, bumps, and matting. Combing your canine's hair gently distributes hair oils, due to this that your dog may additionally have a extra healthy and shinier coat.

Your package want to usually have a comb, scissors, trimmers, and clippers. Depending at the breed, many puppies is probably particularly scared of loud clippers. There are many silent ones in the market specifically created for timid dogs. If you're unsure if your dog will take grooming properly, pass for the silent kit, and don't forget that its belief of this enjoy can constantly be progressed with masses of love, reward, and treats.

Before grooming, make certain your canine is bathed. If your dog regularly performs outside, a weekly bathtub want to suffice. Do no longer bathe your dog extra than as soon as weekly.

If your pup has a thick coat, untangle any knots earlier than you shower it. Use lukewarm water and diluted canine shampoo. Never use cleansing cleaning soap or human shampoo on puppies, no matter the fact that some human beings may also moreover furthermore select to apply horse shampoo for thicker and shinier coats.

With sure breeds, you'll need to put money into a stripping knife. Dogs that do not honestly shed hair will need you to manually strip overgrown and lifeless hair. Make fantastic your canine is cushty with being stripped, otherwise this way may be surprisingly inconvenient for every you and your puppy.

Use nail clippers to hold your canine's nails trimmed. If you don't lessen them often, they'll be greater difficult to reduce the following time you try and do it. Standard scissors paintings outstanding, however I propose the guillotine clipper. If you pass this step, it turns into increasingly hard to your dog to stroll, as their nails will become a curve that pricks at their paws as they float round.

Aside from trimming nails and hair, make sure you often comb your dog to remove any shed hair and maintain its coat smooth and tangle-loose.

Collar or Harness and leash

Although they'll be the maximum apparent ones on the listing, they're without a doubt crucial gadgets irrespective of in that you're preserving your domestic dog till it grows up. Walking your pup can help the 2 of you bond, and could make it emerge as greater snug around humans. And socialize with other puppies.

When it includes collars, ID tags are vital to make sure that your doggy will continuously be diagnosed in case it loses its way. Puppies are usually hyperactive and amusing-loving, so make sure that your leash is a first-rate in shape; otherwise, you could all of sudden lose your grip in case your home canine sees a acquainted neighbor within the distance, or a stray animal it wants to chase.

Optionally, you can get your doggy microchipped, as a way to will can help you discover exactly in which it is. If a microchipped dog ever gets misplaced and a person takes it to a vet, they may use your statistics to touch you and produce your dog once more.

When choosing collars, make certain it's the proper in shape. Collars that are too tight may be extremely uncomfortable in your canine, at the equal time as others can also slip off with out problem. Whatever you select out, make certain which you have extras laying round so that you can with out troubles replace them within the occasion that they wander off.

From my private experience, I decide upon a harness over a collar. This is due to the reality, with a harness, I revel in like I really have higher control over the dog. Also, if the dog unexpectedly pulls, I received't start choking them with a collar, alternatively, I will pull them all over again to its body, using a harness. Harness works flawlessly for all dog sizes; so you don't need to fear if that is probably suitable for yours. Either manner, the final choice is as an awful lot as you.

Carrier

Carriers for large puppies are complex industrial organization, however it's not something that your community doggy keep can't manual you thru. Your domestic canine will likely fit in any plastic carrier, however as your canine grows up, you'll find out yourself switching among large sizes.

You want to normally apprehend the weight and measurements of your dog earlier than you head to a domestic dog shop. Measure your canine from the bottom of its neck to the muse of its tail, then upload some inches for the pinnacle and tail. The height should also be calculated, and the load of your dog contributes to the material you'll select to ensure it's robust enough on your canine's length.

There are plastic and timber carriers, in addition to easy-sided ones. It all is based upon on the way you suggest to use them. If you're for your way to a flight, easy-sided vendors can without issues be located below seats. But if your dog is touring in shipment, ensure the provider is tough, sturdy, and most significantly, properly-ventilated.

If you're using your provider for vet trips, backpack carriers artwork superb for smaller dogs. Bigger dogs can resultseasily be carried to a automobile or taken on public transportation.

Whatever company you buy, ensure it's far durable. If you cheap out in your pet buying spree, you will in all likelihood grow to be repurchasing the whole thing. Bear in thoughts that puppies can without issues escape reasonably-priced material vendors. Dog bed

It doesn't don't forget if you plan to have your dog sleep subsequent to you; your home canine ought to generally have a bed of its very personal. Just like dog homes, dog beds are a part of your high-quality buddy's non-public bubble. And the truth is, dogs will possibly pick out their personal beds over yours.

There are loads of dog beds to be had, and each relies upon on the snoozing fashion of your canine. You can get a sprawler, a burrower, a curler, or a leaner. Shape and layout apart, you want to ensure which you purchase the proper period, which isn't too spacious or too small on your canine however most importantly, purchase a comfortable one.

You'll discover considered one in every of a kind fabrics on the market. Most of them don't make a distinction, so long as you check the label or description of the product and make sure that it's machine-washer-friendly, bearing in thoughts that dog beds will need to be washed often.

Piddle pads and newspapers

Unfortunately, some dogs may be greater hard to educate, and the primary few weeks at your property will possibly be a bit of an adventure. Adding to that is the reality that puppies will be predisposed to leak, so that you'll need to keep your property stocked with all sorts of education pads and line the floors with newspapers until your doggy receives the lay of the land.

When Bella, my now 11-three hundred and sixty five days-vintage Labrador Retriever, changed into a 9 weeks antique domestic dog, I had her drowsing proper subsequent to my bed. She had a lovable pup bed and because of the fact she felt my presence, she didn't even cry from lacking her mummy. I awoke one night with an urge to visit the bathroom, and I generally move in the darkish with out switching the mild on because I knew my condo.

Well, don't do that if you have a new domestic canine inside the room. Bella pooped everywhere within the region and as I walked I stepped proper into this type of unpleasant surprises. Instead of going once more to sleep, I had to wash and clean my rental even as Bella became fortunately napping.

A veterinarian

While that's no longer some aspect you can get at the shop, it's some issue you need to be organized for before you adopt a cutting-edge domestic canine.

Some humans will be predisposed to preserve in mind vet facilities as locations your domestic dog most effective needs to visit while it's ill. Not actual, especially in a puppy's early months. That said, your dog will need to be regularly dewormed and could in the long run must be neutered or spayed, if this hasn't already been completed by using manner of the shelter or breeder. Ask the rescuer/breeder of your puppy if it has already been vaccinated so your vet is privy to what they're handling.

Don't clearly choose the nearest vet to your property. Make extremely good you take a look at opinions in advance than making a decision to consider a vet collectively collectively together with your home canine. If taking your dog to the vet is too much of a problem, domestic visits are also an preference, but can be quite more highly-priced.

Even although getting a dog can also sound like a heartwarming concept, it's moreover a huge duty. So, earlier than you're making the large choice, ensure that your artwork time table permits you to put money into bringing up a puppy. And if that is the primary doggy you private, make certain to the touch your community vet in advance than you carry your canine domestic, to be made aware about the check-u.S.You'll must make to preserve your dog glad and healthful.

Your First Trip

Your first experience along facet your home canine might be the only from the area you take the house dog from. It is a exquisite idea to be organized for that journey but that, of path, relies upon on how a ways you pass and which transport you get. If it's far a long distance(the use of more than 1 hour) and adventure through vehicle, ideally take one greater individual with you. This adventure is probably disturbing to your new domestic canine. It is always better if the house dog is held with the aid of any person else and moreover for safety reasons.

If you haven't any choice to take each other character with you, then it is endorsed you operate a provider or any larger box; that allows you to also do the mission. If you are able to use a seat belt over it for the protection of the domestic canine, that is probably great. Depending on the distance, take some water, bowl, collar, or harness and treats with you. You may want to in all likelihood prevent within the center of the way and stroll your private home canine a piece. If your journey received't take longer than 1 hour, you nearly don't need anything as your domestic dog need to be nicely fed and emptied to final an hour.

What Should The First Day In A New Home Look Like

So you selected your new domestic dog and efficiently transferred it to your own home. What is next?

First of all, the primary day with a present day domestic dog want to be gradual and complete of fun. The dog will probable omit its mom or siblings, so you have to expose them which you're there for them. And what's higher for puppies than playing?

During the number one day, your domestic canine goes to be overly obsessed on everything in its environment. To ensure your domestic dog doesn't get beaten and exhausted through way of all the pride, hold its paws at the ground. You can start through the usage of giving it a mattress and profitable it at the same time as it uses its bed.

Trust is an critical part of a modern day dating, and also you're going to want to earn it. Let your dog discover at its personal tempo and slowly introduce it for your family, or honestly go away it alone in a room and stay up for the domestic dog to come out on its personal. Take care now not to scare your domestic canine with any short movements.

As an extended manner as food goes, make certain you feed your dog frequently and don't overfeed it. You also can mixture dog meals with milk or water. If your canine doesn't stop its meal, don't worry, because it's regular for a younger pup to play with its food as an opportunity of truly eating it. You also can choose wet meals, as lengthy because it's not canned.

Tips And Tricks To Avoid Puppy's Homesickness

If you have ever professional homesickness, you likely might not need to wish that on all people else. Your pup may additionally moreover sense homesick within the night time but always doesn't should.

I continuously had my puppies inside the course of my mattress just so they could feel my presence. Luckily, they not often cried and it could be one of the examined recipes to save you homesickness. I am frequently very eager to endorse this method to all and sundry who has supplied a today's domestic dog.

Puppies usually cry inside the night on the equal time as all settles down and they start to bypass over their mom. A appropriate trick I moreover locate powerful is placing a warm bottle of water within the puppy's bed. That bottle will imitate the warmth of her mom.

If you consider you studied that dogs can be homesick definitely at night time time, you may be amazed. Puppies can cry in some unspecified time within the destiny of the day too. If your home dog suggests any forms of homesickness and disappointment, you will probable restore that with the aid of going through this listing.

1. Always make certain your domestic canine has somewhere cushty to sleep and relaxation. Buy a canine mattress and place it somewhere comfortable. Your dog need to in no way be forced to sleep with you on your mattress, but if you'd want to do that, make sure that the dog generally has a safe area to retreat to in the occasion that they want it.

2. Never cross too far from home with out your dog. Many puppies experience homesickness whilst they'll be separated from domestic, and this isn't probable to trade. As you are the chief of the p.C. Now, your domestic dog will look as plenty as you as their god/goddess. The greater time you spend together along facet your dog, the better. As you have got were given already positioned, the touch among the 2 of you helps you bond better.

3. Remember that dogs are like children too, and that they also can enjoy homesickness and need reassurance. Give your home canine lots of hobby, with hundreds of hugs and cuddles (ultimately, it's far all about love). This need to help every you and your domestic canine experience better, further to ensuring that there can be masses much less of a chance for strain for the animal.

four. Try playing track within the records on the equal time as you are out of the house. This will assist hold your dog occupied, thinking, and curious about what one of a kind humans is probably there.

five. Remember, puppies are very touchy and can enjoy human feelings. No rely extensive range how dissatisfied you're, your canine wishes reassurance from you at a time like this. Don't argue or don't combat inside the the front of your home dog. It is similar to with a human infant. Try to preserve the electricity easy and resolve any problem a ways from anyone else. When your pup shows symptoms of stress, smile and guarantee them that the whole lot is amazing.

Wow, another economic disaster in the back of you. You determined all you need to put together in advance than bringing the pup domestic, you found about a way to nicely get the domestic dog home, and what the primary day want to be like. You moreover understand a way to save you or address a home canine's homesickness.

Your pup is now home with you and this is an superb time first of all education. In the following economic disaster, you can studies everything approximately the paintings of nice reinforcement and its importance. You will discover considered one of a kind forms of canine schooling and I will teach you over 10 easy instructions in your domestic canine, so you can start raising an exquisite pup companion. So go with the flow in advance and flip to the subsequent net net page.

Chapter 7: Puppy Is Home, Training Is On

Now which you understand how to be the sturdy percentage leader that your domestic canine desires, it's time which you have a have a look at the significance of splendid reinforcement, that could be a manner you may use to educate your doggy number one obedience. Since this e-book is set elevating and training your home canine with love, the training technique of first-rate reinforcement has been tested to be type and very powerful.

Training with exceptional reinforcement is rooted within the antique announcing 'You can seize more flies with honey than with vinegar.' Your pup wants to please their alpha, and using that as a training method makes lifestyles much less complex and loads extra high-quality for every of you!

Art of Positive Reinforcement

Positive reinforcement is sincerely an art work. It combines a mild manner to train your private home dog with precision timing. Positive reinforcement rewards a dog for behaving within the expected manner, but refrains from the usage of loud voices or physical approaches in any other case. There's no real 'punishment' for awful behavior. Punishment is terrible reinforcement. If it's now not the favored behavior, it's disregarded as a superb deal as possible. Attention, even lousy hobby, reinforces terrible behavior. Treats, interest, and snuggling can handiest be done via giving the conduct that turn out to be preferred via the alpha.

There is a stable scientific basis to why satisfactory reinforcement can be very powerful as a education method. Dogs are creatures of addiction. They price ordinary and look for patterns in their every day activities. They discover about their companions and surroundings in the identical way a infant or infant does—thru way of repetition.

This manner that if a domestic canine is constantly rewarded for behaving in a terrific way, it'll hold following that behavioral pattern till it becomes a addiction. Therefore, in the long run, you may not must praise your house canine for correct conduct on every occasion they carry out it, because it absolutely turns into their 2d nature to behave that manner. Positive reinforcement is a humane and non-threatening way to educate any preferred behaviors. It furthermore shows dogs and puppies alike that their human circle of relatives, and especially their alpha, may be relied on, and that prevents strain and allows them to experience secure.

Confidence, and now not worry, is instilled along the coolest conduct that form each time an proprietor makes use of fantastic schooling techniques. Canines are very practical and first-rate reinforcement makes them use that intelligence. They are challenged to figure subjects out and now and again you could nearly see the wheels turning in their heads.

It is essential to phrase that dogs are first rate at studying frame language, so controlling your bodily expressions is critical. It's a natural form of communication for them. Dogs use ear and tail role, further to complete body stance, to permit every fantastic apprehend friendliness, challenge, willingness to combat, protectiveness, and % position. Don't be amazed if your domestic dog is going stomach up—the location of submission—once they meet a person or some one-of-a-kind canine. They are really acknowledging that they definitely outrank them and they collect it! Make positive that your frame language is high high-quality as a manner to ship them the appropriate messages.

Other favored behaviors can be achieved the equal manner. If sitting gets a smile and a deal with and jumping up doesn't get something, guess whose butt will start hitting the floor frequently! When you begin residence-education, additionally start education the crucial commands, especially 'take a seat.' Make that domestic dog take a seat right down to get a cope with, sit down down right down to get their food, and sit down in advance than playtime or petting. In a percentage, not some factor is unfastened; rewards are earned. Be the alpha who dreams and rewards ideal conduct.

When education your home canine, if there may be an low fee situation and command you deliver it, constantly impose it. Don't genuinely bypass that with a smile and hug your pup. That is simply reinforcing their disobedience and you are losing apprehend in the domestic canine's eyes. You, as a leader of a %, the alpha ought to be expert and that excellent takes area if your domestic dog listens to you while you need it.

One of the maximum vital schooling you will want is leash education. If you don't want to be dragged behind your dog, get a leash tangled among your legs and jumping the pup from one side to another, then preserve on studying. Let's have a check how to use the art work of high exquisite reinforcement while education your private home dog on a leash.

Indoor Potty Training

An indoor dog potty may be very useful on your circle of relatives, specially with a modern-day home dog. While you continue to want to educate your dog to use a rest room outside, indoor toilet solutions regardless of the fact that have an area for the duration of sticky conditions like dwelling in a excessive-upward thrust rental, now not having too much time on hand, or no longer being physical capable of walking your doggy every 2-3 hours or sincerely cold climate.

Either way, potty schooling can help you treatment some of those troubles, however should no longer be the number one manner to teach your puppy to excrete. There are many styles of canine potties from fake grass to self-cleansing potty pads. It all relies upon on what you pick and how much you are willing to spend. Dogs don't like doing their enterprise in a place they sleep. It is against their herbal instinct. However, as a pup, this will take some time for them to apprehend what is their territorium and what isn't, and this is why indoor potty training makes it feasible.

How to do Indoor Potty Training

Puppies amplify their behavior right away, so displaying them in which to move and what to do is the fastest way to achievement.

Your domestic dog will create a super affiliation with doing their commercial organization out of doors, however in this situation moreover indoors in the event that they have the urgency however can't pass outdoor.

1.   Create a preferred potty area in a wonderful spot than in which the puppy sleeps

2.   Introduce a potty mat in your doggy with the aid of way of being there with them, making notable establishments thru play and treats

three.   Wait till they excrete

four.   Praise them with love, and praise them with a address

Puppies usually don't must excrete right away when you are there with them however recall, that puppies are notably intuitive. Maybe your home canine will get it proper the primary time, perhaps it's going to take the time however in the long run, they'll create a amazing affiliation with going to excrete in a favored vicinity. As I stated, don't take it as the precept solution. Your puppy wishes to be walked and socialized, however, this solution can though be in hand if your home dog urgently desires to cross potty right away.

Leash Training

Loose leash on foot

New puppy will be pulling you on a leash and it'd be a miracle if it did no longer. Leash pulling takes vicinity at the same time as your canine is happy and wants to flow into faster than you. It receives a chunk difficult to trap up with the speed of your canine because it definitely possesses a quicker pace than people.

It is vital to teach your domestic dog to keep leash manners as it may get annoying for you. It may additionally lead your dog to pull tough and let loose, this is the ultimate factor you need.

By training your canine to prevent immoderate leash pulling, you could have the comfort of taking walks at a sustained tempo, whilst your canine will pause collectively with you or look beforehand in your permission to alleviate itself at a selected spot.

I want to provide you a few effective recommendations and suggestions for this schooling, an excellent way to help you hold your doggy underneath regular manage on the equal time as on a leash.

Get the right accessories

Uninformed dog proprietors would possibly in truth purchase a leash with out expertise the types available, and the effect it would have on their dogs. Get more information at the form of collar, harness, and leash that might be suitable on your canine, consistent with its period and breed, or ask for assist. I recommend the usage of a ordinary leash and a no-pull dog harness if your house dog has a bent to have this trouble.

Use rewards

Occasional rewards inside the form of treats or a favourite toy are beneficial in garnering your puppy's interest. Use it at the equal time as you educate your pup on a leash. Walking one step at a time—at the same time as keeping your pup's interest the usage of a reward—will make it magically adapt its motion to you.

The command you operate for this kind of scenario is "With me". If a domestic dog maintains on foot proper next to your left leg, maintain encouraging them with the resource of announcing "nicely boy/female". Show manage and say "no" even as it insists on transferring ahead by means of tugging at the string. Once it calms down, reward it and offer a deal with. This will slowly construct an instinct in it to have a study your orders, especially on the equal time as on a leash.

Remember, in education, it is continually higher to keep it shorter than longer. I will as an alternative train my home canine a couple of instances a day for five mins than mocking them 1/2-hour in a row. Firstly, it's miles however a domestic dog and has heaps to find out on this international. Secondly, a domestic canine will become bored because of the fact the span of its interest is brief.

Important tip: Practice a long way from people. The extra humans and gadgets, the bigger distraction it's far on your pup. You need to educate your house dog somewhere secluded if feasible so that you can get their most attention.

Stand although and exchange course

If your doggy continues on pulling, use techniques like repute nonetheless or converting direction. When your canine starts offevolved pulling, be glued to the spot for some time and then flip around to walk in the opposite path. This will make it apprehend that its conduct is unacceptable, and that it doesn't get what it dreams thru pulling.

Pulling on the leash is a behavioral problem so that it will take time to enhance, so be affected person and regular in schooling. Some dogs are substantially more energetic than others, so it might be a exceptional concept to hotel to professional education if this is the case together with your domestic canine. No matter number quantity what your precise case is, although, recall that pulling greater tough at the leash in go once more will simplest be counterproductive, so hold a non violent and assertive mind-set and don't try and treatment this problem with muscle energy.

Another manner to use the artwork of satisfactory reinforcement is clicker training. Clicker training is an non-compulsory technique with the intention to art work for maximum puppies, and the clean idea is to replace treats for clicks, and it works first rate while transitioning your dog from address rewards into click on rewards.

Clicker Training

For many dogs, a clicker is a terrific way to teach them. Small and much less highly-priced, clickers artwork by means of manner of taking snap shots your canine's interest with an audible sound. You'll use the clicker with a voice command, and in the event that they do the proper issue then you virtually'll deliver your domestic dog a address.

Benefits of a Clicker

This method allows to stop your canine from being relying at the treats and in spite of the fact that be aware of you. You received't have to name or yell at your domestic dog, and they may be able to pay interest the clicker at an prolonged range. This makes it less complex to educate them in your voice, and your home canine will start to look to you for leadership extra quick.

Simply press the clicker's button at the same time as your doggy does what you need them to do and follow the press with a excessive first-class reward, including a small cope with or an enthusiastic, encouraging domestic canine, a scratch in the back of the ears, and a "best boy/female!" verbal reinforcement.

Step through Step Process

Here is a step-through-step on how to teach your dog the use of a clicker. Make sure you get a clicker that works properly to get began out.

1. Use a Command: You must start out with a intention in thoughts. What behavior do you need to intention first? One of the great ones to reason is "sit down". Raise your hand up

with a deal with visible in it and tell your doggy to sit down.

2. Give a Treat: Make positive that you offer the deal with as fast as they may be within the right characteristic. You don't need to have too prolonged of a delay or this will harm the affiliation way.

three. Repeat: Do it all once more, and ensure which you use the same movement together with the same tone.

4. Vary Reward: Do it a few more instances, and while you do you'll want to differ the reward you're giving them. Sometimes, actually puppy them, once in a while say "correct boy/lady!" and on occasion use a cope with.

5. Clicker: Once the puppy has already made the association, that's even as the clicker is to be had in. Repeat the technique of asking them to sit down down, then press the clicker's button, and look at the click with a tremendous reward, alongside side a small

address or an encouraging puppy. They don't apprehend what the brand new noise is but.

6. Repeat: This time you're going to tell your dog to sit down down, maintaining the clicker and cope with over their head. Remember to click on on it as you convey it up. Give them a deal with. Keep repeating.

7. Clicker: Use truely the clicker, and if your dog sits provide them a deal with. You don't must use phrases now.

Make great that you in no manner teach your canine in a manner wherein the clicker truely receives their interest. You need to assign it to a certain command. Keep in thoughts that a few dogs will have a look at slower than others, and you could't anticipate your domestic canine to learn how to reply to the clicker in handiest an afternoon or .

When you train your canine every specific command with the clicker, then you definately without a doubt want to differ the click. One-click on on on can be "sit", however fast clicks will need to be something like "lie down". However, in case you want to function every exceptional including "stay," you could use both 3 speedy clicks or sluggish clicks. If you have got a difficult time together together with your doggy not in search of to pay interest, strive giving them a destroy. Just like kids, they now and again want to exit for recess, and school can't be each single day.

Essential Commands

There are many special theories approximately a way to train a pup. Some humans bear in mind in firmness and strict instructions that include effects. Other colleges of idea will tell you that offering rewards for proper behavior and putting off rewards for lousy behavior is the exceptional way to teach a puppy. The fine direction of motion actually relies upon on your dog and the animal's precise man or woman. Some puppies can be interested in appealing you and others will not in reality care what you think. The tremendous manner to technique obedience education together with your home canine is to apply regular exercise. Remember that puppies are young and active, so hold your schooling commands quick and make sure they will be now not hungry or tired.

"Heel"

Teaching your doggy the manner to heel is important, in particular while there are unique puppies spherical, or people that your canine also can need to leap on without invitation. When you command your dog to heel, the dog will sit down by using the usage of the usage of your issue quietly until launched. This is a difficult factor for puppies to examine, especially in view that they may be so lively and curious by using manner of nature. This command can be very crucial at the same time as you want to move the street or virtually clearly keep your house dog through the use of your facet.

You can use this command to make your domestic canine much less aggravating of sounds out of doors your own home. Try doing this exercise on the same time as traversing a busy sidewalk. Be vigilant at this factor and ensure they heel whenever they experience too curious. Stop strolling within the event that they do not be aware about you.

The key to this part of domestic canine schooling is of direction treats. Start with the resource of reputation together collectively together with your pup on a leash and maintain some treats inside the hand that isn't always protective the leash. The home dog desires to understand the command, so inform your dog to heel. Once they sit down down down however subsequent to you for about 5 seconds, deliver the dog a address. Then, take 5 steps forward and permit your canine to comply with. Say the phrase "heel" and anticipate your doggy to sit down down subsequent to you. Reward with a deal with. Continue doing this so your pup is conscious. The dog will associate your moves and phrases with the anticipated behaviors.

Once this is correctly finished within the same area, introduce some wonderful people and distractions. You might also moreover revel in like you are beginning the machine all once more, however it surely is exceptional because your puppy can be aware the ones different people or bouncing balls or transferring vehicles. Repeat the way with the treats till your dog is obedient and able to heel on command.

"Sit"

Use a hand gesture with the "sit down" command. The right hand gesture for this is the use of the index finger pointing up and inside the direction of your property canine. Get your home canine's interest by using way of pronouncing their call, saying the command, and on the equal time acting the gesture. Once finished correctly, praise immediately. This is my favored technique, preferably over a Clicker. This approach applies for each unmarried command. Sooner or later you can find out that you don't need to speak anymore. You will genuinely use hand gestures and your canine will concentrate.

For dogs who find out it tough to recognize the "sit down" command, you could faucet their rump to convey attention to that body element. Lightly push all the way down to encourage a sitting function and then say the command "sit down". Use this method sparingly as your home dog could probable associate this touching movement as a praise. It need to most effective be used to get an preliminary response. Teaching your own home canine to sit down down down isn't always complex, and the canine will apprehend what you want at the same time as you praise it with treats and bodily display the animal what you expect. Stand within the front of your puppy and keep your hand above its head with a deal with in it. They will appearance up at it. Use your one of a kind hand to softly push down on their hindquarters until they're in a sitting function.

At the equal time, on the identical time as no matter the fact that retaining the treat, say "sit" in a non violent but business enterprise voice. Once they may be capable of keep the location, provide the puppy the deal with. Keep repeating this motion until the home dog is capable of positioned itself proper proper right into a sitting feature without your steerage. Ultimately, the puppy can be capable of sit down down with out your help. This is specially useful for greeting conditions whilst you're introducing your canine to new people. Tell the puppy to sit down and while that occurs, be coming near near with the address.

Once your private home canine is aware what you want with out you physical pushing them down, carry out the command status in the front of them, commanding verbally, and accompanying them with a gesture.

If your pup rapid loses the training you have mastered, absolutely begin once more. You would probably word your puppy jumps on people even as they come into your private home or runs after kids in the network. Give the command to take a seat, and if the dog does no longer pay attention, cross all over again to the fundamentals with the address and the bodily lowering of your dog into the sitting characteristic.

"Stay"

The right hand gesture for this command is with an open palm pointing within the route of the domestic dog.

Teaching a home canine to live might be a hint difficult as it's counter-intuitive to a domestic dog, who desires to discover and soar and sniff and bark. First, designate a niche in which you want your dog to live. That might be a dog bed, a nook of the room, or a specific region that maintains the home canine far from whatever you are doing.

Give the command to "stay" and use your hand gesture at the equal time. Continue to duplicate the word "stay" so your pup is privy to to companion that word with the command. Praise the home canine while you get the obedience you are seeking out and the dog remains at the spot you've got got precise. Wait 10 seconds and reward your doggy with a cope with.

"Come"

The proper hand gesture for this command is with an open palm placed at the middle of your chest.

Puppies generally want to come back at the same time as they're called. They need to realise what you are as a good buy as and they may be going to be eager to be close to you and be part of something you're doing. However, it could be tough to get your house canine to come lower back if the doggy is preoccupied with something else.

Maybe the home dog is digging within the out of doors or stalking a squirrel or honestly enthusiastic about the fragrance on a few random vehicle's tires. The trick is to train the dog that coming to you is the awesome preference that could ever be made. When you call your doggy's call and your little friend comes going for walks over, shower that dog with praise, love, and treats. With that kind of affection and fine reinforcement, your home canine will in no manner want to overlook the possibility to return to you on the same time as called.

For education functions, name your home dog from one room to each different. Stand in the kitchen, at the same time as your puppy is in the dwelling room, and make contact with the canine through the use of call and use the hand gesture on the equal time. When your domestic canine comes on foot, get excited, pet them and provide a cope with. When the doggy is capable of understand that coming at the same time as referred to as technique only exceptional matters, they'll obey proper now.

Pro Tip: Some puppies might be hesitant to head returned as they could see you as a large, tall man or woman which can in all likelihood sign a capacity hazard. If for a few aspect motive your domestic dog wouldn't take note of this command, attempt to bend for your knees and reduce yourself. Then carry out the command with the hand gesture. This way you appear as a lesser danger to the domestic dog psychologically, since you are smaller and shorter. That need to work perfectly.

"Lie Down"

The right hand gesture for this command is with an open palm pointing closer to the ground whilst you start at a degree of your decrease chest and circulate down to the quantity of your navel.

Training your property dog to lie down is similar to the manner you knowledgeable the dog to sit down. Find a gap that you need the canine to companion with lying down. That will in all likelihood be a dog bed or a mat. Pat the region at the side of your hand and say the phrases "lie down." If you need to, lower your canine's body to the ground so the pup is aware of what mendacity down way. Reward the very last act with a deal with as everyday. Keep training until your domestic dog receives it. Your doggy could probable have a number of its very personal mind approximately in which the super places to lie down are. Respect that intuition and teach the doggy to lie down inside the locations that they appear maximum snug.

"Stand"

It is the opposite of the "lie down" command. The right hand gesture for this command is with an open palm pointing in the course of the sky whilst you begin on the volume of your navel and skip as masses as the quantity of your lower chest.

This command is used at the same time as your home canine is lying at the floor and you want them to rise up. Or might be used at the same time as your home dog sits and that is the command that tells them to face another time. Very clean, use any form of reward on the identical time because the command is finished correctly.

"Take It"

There isn't any hand gesture required while appearing this command. You and your domestic canine may additionally seem in a scenario wherein you could through this command inspire your doggy to "take it". This is probably taking some thing out of your hand, or taking a few factor from the ground. Easy, simply maintain speaking for your house canine, sooner or later they will apprehend.

"Drop it"

There is not any hand gesture required at the same time as appearing this command each. However, that is a completely critical command. A situation wherein your dog chews a few element which may be unstable to them whilst swallowing, isn't any fun. "Drop it" may be applied in all kinds of conditions. It commands that regardless of the domestic dog has in its mouth, it have to drop it now! You can teach this command with a chewing toy. Optionally, you can factor your finger and call the ground in which you want the item to be dropped.

"No"

The proper gesture for this command is easy. Your head transferring from proper to left will do. As you'll gesture to a human, this is the same scenario.

Puppies do now not understand right from incorrect and in case you want them to save you chewing, biting, jumping, or barking, you want to teach them to understand the word "no." When your house dog does a few factor you do now not like, say the word "no" in a organisation, loud voice. If the home dog obeys, praise with a cope with.